COVID-19 AND THE VIRUS THAT SHOOK THE WORLD

MIRIAM CALLEJA

OPPIAN

Published by Oppian Press
Helsinki, Finland

ISBN 978-951-877-140-4

oppian.fi

CONTENTS

INTRODUCTION TO VIRUSES

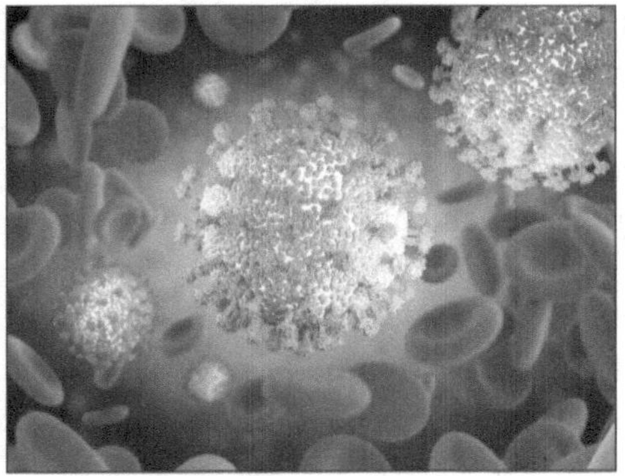

Viruses are the most abundant organic beings on earth. They are present everywhere within our environment as well as inside us. However, they do not perform all the functions we consider vital for a biological entity to be classified as a life form. They have no cellular structure and they lack most components of cells. They cannot make their own energy, nor grow without a host cell. Once a virus enters a host cell, though, it can take over and use the cell to make more copies of itself. It depends on the host cell for energy and the raw materials for this to happen. A virus cannot sustain itself.

Viruses are principally composed of a nucleic acid core, an outer protein coating, and sometimes an outer protein envelope. The nucleic acid core can be composed of either DNA or RNA, never both. Viruses may also have other proteins, for example, enzymes.

Viruses can be thought of as parasitic since they use hosts, be it plants, birds, insects, or mammals (including humans) to replicate and ensure their continued existence. They can only replicate by using a host's cells and thus thrive via infection. Although they are not living, they can affect the behaviour of their host. Viruses are not always harmful to their host and may exist within cells in a dormant state or at a very slow rate of replication, seemingly undetected by the immune system.

Viruses are and have been, an important factor in transferring genes between different species, and thus in the increase of genetic diversity. One theory suggests that the arrival of the nucleus in life forms on earth may have come about through a persistent DNA virus.

Prokaryotes, such as bacteria, are organisms whose cells do not have membrane-bound organelles. These are small, generally microscopic, and relatively simple cells surrounded by a membrane and cell wall containing a circular strand of DNA. The nucleus is a part of the cell that differentiates eukaryotes from prokaryotes. Eukaryotic cells are more complex due to their specialised organelles, and they generally belong to multicellular organisms. In eukaryotes, the DNA is linear and found within a nucleus. The general consensus is that eukaryotes evolved from prokary-otes, possibly via the actions of a type of virus called the retrovirus. Some evidence supports this theory, but the exact steps involved in this process are not confirmed.

Viruses are the microscopic particles responsible for some of the most threatening diseases, including influenza, smallpox, ebola, and rabies. Due to their ever-changing nature, they have been difficult to cate-gorise and to understand.

What coronaviruses are

Coronaviruses (CoVs) are a large family of viruses that infect humans, animals, and birds. In both animals and humans, they cause respiratory and intestinal infec-tions. The respiratory illnesses can range from the common cold to more severe and acute respiratory diseases.

Coronaviruses are named after their appearance, with 'corona' meaning 'crown' or 'halo' in Latin. These viruses have a characteristic spherical shape with crown-like spikes on their surface and measure around 100-160nm in diameter.

Each coronavirus' genetic material comprises posi-tive-sense single-stranded RNA (or (+)ssRNA). This means that the positive-sense RNA genome of the virus can use the host cell's ribosomes to directly translate RNA into protein. Ribosomes are in all living cells. They serve as a site of biological protein synthesis by linking amino acids in the order defined by the messenger RNA. Each virus body contains a single-stranded positive-sense RNA genome that interacts with the nucleoprotein, measuring 27-32 kb.

They are on the larger side with viruses and also have the largest genome in comparison with all other RNA viruses. This RNA genome is found inside a helical nucleocapsid protein and further surrounded by another membrane coating called an envelope. Three different proteins are incorporated within the viral envelope: Membrane (M), Envelope (E) and Spike (S) proteins. The M and E proteins are associated with assembling the virus. The S protein moderates the virus infiltration into the host cells.

Coronaviruses that affect human health are of the family *Coronaviridae* subfamily *Coronavirinae*. There are four main sub-groupings of human coronaviruses - alpha, beta, gamma, and delta. Among these genera included in this subfamily, *Alphacoronavirus* and *Betacoronavirus* are the ones which interest clinical virologists. Some of these viruses were first identified and described in the 1960s, and until this day, we know of seven coronaviruses that can affect the human population. Four of these seven coronaviruses commonly affect people around the world.

The relatively newer (or 'novel') coronaviruses that have infected people are MERS-CoV, SARS-CoV and SARS-CoV-2 (which causes COVID-19). Until the appearance of Severe Acute Respiratory Syndrome (SARS) in 2002 coronaviruses were thought of as minor pathogens for humans. Until then, they were only linked to the common cold or mild respiratory symptoms affecting immunocompromised people and rarely exhibiting severe infections in the elderly or the very young.

Coronaviruses are zoonotic, meaning they can be

passed between animals and humans. Until the 21st century, coronaviruses were not considered highly pathogenic to the human race. When the outbreak of severe acute respiratory syndrome (SARS) occurred in 2002 and 2003 in the Guangdong province of China, the first severe infections were seen. Before that only mild infections had been observed, and these mostly occurred in those with compromised immune systems. It was, therefore, SARS that put coronaviruses in the spotlight and highlighted the need for experts to continue learning more about this family of viruses.

Ten years after the outbreak of SARS, another coronavirus was identified, which was also highly pathogenic, and this was the Middle East Respiratory Syndrome coronavirus (MERS-CoV).

Both SARS and MERS were studied extensively, and this has led to a better understanding of the origin, composition, and behaviour of coronaviruses. On the basis of sequence databases obtained from these and several other types of coronaviruses, it has been established that all human coronaviruses have animal origins.

HOW ZOONOSIS HAPPENS?

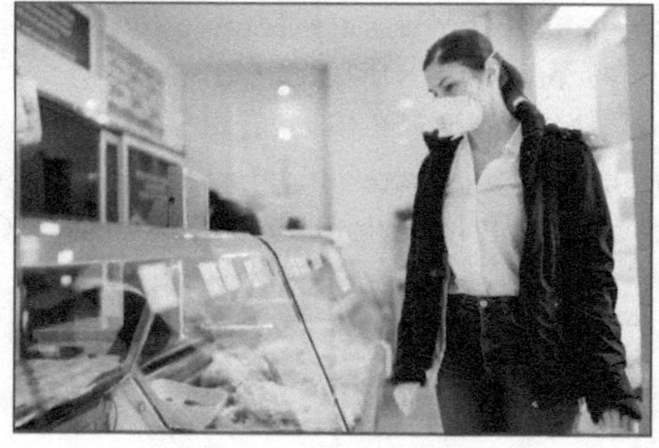

The word zoonosis comes from the Greek terms for: ζῷον *zoon* "animal" and νόσος *nosos* "sickness".

Zoonosis is a type of infectious disease that passes from an animal or insect to a human. These can be viruses, bacteria, fungi, and parasites. They do not always necessarily infect the animal. Sometimes more than one type of animal can be involved in this transmission so that one animal can be an intermediary transmitting the zoonotic microbe between an animal and a human.

Zoonotic diseases are common throughout the world. It is estimated that around 60% of known infectious diseases in people can be spread from animals and that three-quarters of new and emerging diseases in humans come from animals. Zoonosis can be of two types: either direct or indirect. Even though most infectious diseases originated in non-human animals, only diseases that consistently involve non-human to human transmission can be classified as direct zoonosis.

In direct zoonosis, the disease is transmitted directly from the animal to a human through media such as air, or via saliva or bites.

Direct zoonosis can happen in various ways because of the close connection between people and some animals. These can include:

- Direct contact

Coming into contact with bodily fluids or excrements such as blood, saliva, mucus, faeces, and urine. It can also include petting and touching the animals or any interaction that causes the animal to scratch or bite.

- Indirect contact

Being in areas and touching areas where animals live or pass through, as well as objects contaminated with viruses, bacteria, fungi, or parasites, e.g., animal barns, pet food or water dishes, chicken coops, plants, and soil.

- Vector-borne

Getting bitten by a tick or flea or an insect such as a mosquito.

- Foodborne

By eating or drinking something unsafe such as unpasteurized milk or cheese made with such milk.

Other food that has come into contact with faeces and not washed well, such as raw fruits and vegetables, can also be a source of zoonotic disease. Undercooked meat or other contaminated foods such as eggs that have come from an infected source can also cause infection.

• Waterborne

Coming into contact or drinking water contaminated with the faeces of a diseased animal can also be a source of infectious disease.

Zoonotic diseases can be global, or they may be limited to certain parts of the world. However, as rates of worldwide travel increases, markets globalise, and humans keep encroaching on the natural habitat of animals, the numbers and range of zoonotic disease may increase. There are also several known coronaviruses circulating in animals not yet transmitted to and infected humans.

When a new coronavirus crosses over to human hosts and can then be transmitted from human to human, this poses problems due to its novel nature. Since they have not been exposed to this virus before, they cannot be protected by their natural immunity and vaccines against it are not available. The mutations can rapidly lead to outbreaks, epidemics, and eventually pandemics. This happened in the previous outbreaks of SARS and MERS.

Aside from being a public health problem, zoonosis may also cause obstacles in the efficient production of food of animal origin for human consumption and in the international trade of animal products.

How does zoonosis happen?

. . .

Although this happens rarely, viruses that usually only affect certain animal species can undergo a mutation that creates new strains that can cross over to human hosts. Some examples of this are anthrax, plague, Lyme disease, rabies, typhus, and West Nile fever. Not all mutations are 'bad' mutations that can lead to zoonosis and interspecies transfer. Viruses of the RNA kind are less stable in their multiplication and thus 'mistakes' in this cloning of the RNA is more likely than with DNA types.

Several key factors have been observed to aid the zoonotic virus spillover to a range of taxonomically different animal vectors, which can infect humans and cause human-to-human transmission. It was also found that wild animals were significantly more likely to facilitate this transfer as compared to domesticated species. However, it was found that domestic animals play a central role in cross-species transmission.

Historically it has been those with occupational exposure to animals affected by zoonotic virus spillover, such as hunters, veterinarians, researchers, laboratory workers, wildlife management in zoos or sanctuaries. Rodent hosts were often implicated in the transmission of zoonotic by indirect contact in and around human homes.

The situation has changed as humans encroach on wild animal habitats more and more. Certain circumstances such as 'wet markets' for wildlife create an unnatural situation where animals that would not normally mix in nature are caged and undergo stressful situations before being sold or killed in the same space. Animals kept in cramped and unhygienic situations are obviously stressed and a low immune system caused by this stress makes them susceptible to disease. This creates a favourable opportunity for a virus to cross species via animal to animal contact, contact with blood or faeces, sharing of food, or via vectors such as mosquitoes or fleas.

We think that the virus has one aim - to spread from host to host so its continued existence is assured. To this end, attaining the capability of spreading from human-to-human is a desirable feature. Another desirable feature is that of having host plasticity, that is being able to survive in, and replicate in, a number of hosts of different taxonomic orders.

A sudden appearance of such a new agent can quickly cause an epidemic if the agent is particularly virulent, as with the HIV and the AIDS epidemic.

Diseases that have been eradicated, such as smallpox, are typically not zoonotic diseases. And therefore do not have an animal reservoir. The animal reservoir is what can lead to recurrent outbreaks of a disease, and it is what makes these diseases so unpredictable and difficult to avoid and handle.

IS THE NEW CORONAVIRUS ONE OF MANY TO COME?

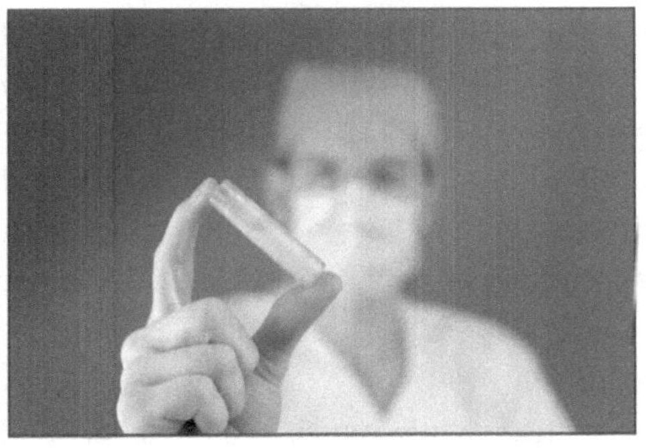

The virosphere is defined as a collection of places where viruses can be found on the planet. Even though they are primarily thought of as infectious agents, viruses have a role to play in the world, and many functions inside and outside of us depend on them. They play a part in our immune system and in the ecosystems of land and sea, they regulate climate and affect the evolution of all species.

When the virus that causes COVID-19, which we

now know as SARS-CoV-2, was first discovered, it came under the limelight and to the forefront of our attention. However, scientists have long known, discussed, and written papers about the millions, perhaps trillions, of species of viruses waiting to be identified - hopefully not as this latest one was.

Scientists have recently used Artificial Intelligence (AI) in their search for the identification of viral genes from samples of water, mud, blood, soil, seawater, and other materials. They are in a phase where the discovery of a diversity of new viruses is growing exponentially, but describing new viruses is a costly and time-consuming task.

Taking SARS-CoV-2 as an example, first, this was isolated and examined - it was found to have the distinctive crown of proteins typical of coronaviruses. This was followed by a gene sequencing conducted by virologists to try to determine more of its properties. Since it was found to be genetically similar to the virus that caused SARS known as SARS-CoV, the new virus was classified as a coronavirus and named SARS-CoV-2.

The struggle with figuring out classes and kingdoms of viruses is that they exchange genes with other species, making it hard to select groups. Their existence is dynamic and this interchange may even sometimes make them harder to fight.

While priority was given to this virus, there are hundreds of thousands more awaiting naming and classification and far more waiting to be identified. Many viruses infecting animals, plants, fungi, and protozoans may never cross over to the human species. Yet learning about various viruses and the way they act may be the key to a better understanding of this virosphere, and may lead experts to come up with new ways to combat the ones that become a threat.

HOW DO CORONAVIRUSES SPREAD?

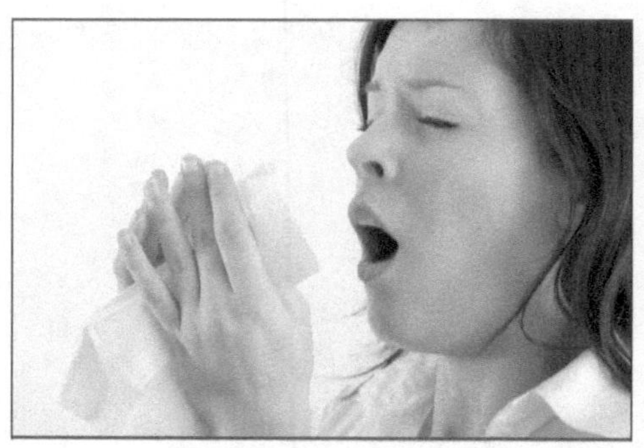

The basic reproductive ratio - known as R_0 - is the projected number of secondary infections resulting from a single individual during their infectious period, presuming the population they encounter is susceptible to the particular disease. It is a parameter fundamental to the study of epidemiology and to the understanding of pathogen dynamics within a host. R_0 is used to understand and predict how an infection will spread within a population.

If patient number 1 has been infected with

COVID-19 and he is going about his day normally, the estimation is that he can infect 2-3 people, this is the R_0 of COVID-19. If these 3 infected people do the same, 9 people could get infected. When these 9 people interact normally in society, they could infect 3 people each, quickly bringing the number of infected people to 27. This is an exponential rise. However, if social distancing is in place, the spread would be much slower. This is especially important since infection with COVID-19 may take up to 14 days to result in symptoms, and sometimes there will be very mild symptoms or none at all. Infected people can spread the virus during the whole period of infection.

The infection will spread if patient 1 coughs or sneezes near these people and they breathe these droplets in, or if he releases droplets onto surfaces these people then touch. Once infected surfaces are touched, these new people are not automatically infected. Infection will happen if they touch their face and, in particular, their mucous membranes without having washed their hands well. Infection may also happen if they take an object containing these droplets into their home and the object is touched by another member of the same household who touches their face. SARS-CoV-2 can exist for a limited amount of time on certain surfaces, with the amount of time varying depending on the material in question.

Using the same example above, if just one of the first 3 infected people practices social distancing and proper hygiene practices we already see a difference, as the next batch of infected patients would be expected to total to 6 instead of 9, then 18 instead of 27. From this, the more people practice social distancing, the less likely it is for the infection to spread.

The comparison with influenza is not fair since there is a way to get protected from influenza with a yearly flu shot. Thus there is the presumption that not all encounters hold the potential of contagion. In addition to that, we know more about the progression of disease with the flu and have a number of established treatment options to stop the disease from progressing to a severe state. Even though thousands of people around the world die of the flu each year, we can prevent many more from dying. In contrast, there is yet no vaccine, herd immunity, or established treatment or cure in place against COVID-19. This should be done only for the sake of understanding the concepts in play in this situation.

When comparing influenza to COVID-19, we see that influenza has an R_0 of 1, so each infected patient will spread influenza to 1 other person. If one of these patients practices social distancing soon enough, then the spread will stop at that patient, and as the previous patients get better, the number of infected people from that thread of infection will go back to zero.

However, it is also known that influenza has a short series interval, making the possible contagion to other people start earlier upon infection compared to COVID-19. This is the time between the onset of symptoms in primary and secondary cases. That means that using the examples above, it would take a longer time for the second wave of infection to occur, i.e., for the hypothesised 3 patients to start showing symptoms. Symptomatic patients are more likely to spread disease through droplets, as they will be sneezing and coughing, thus aiding droplet expulsion.

. . .

Politics of spread

There are a number of methods that experts use to determine the value of R_0, and in the past, these methods have been used to study demographics, the spread of vector-borne diseases such as malaria, and to study infections directly transmitted between humans.

When R_0 is smaller than 1, then the individual with the infection will spread the disease, on average, to less than one new individual. That means that infection might not occur at all, and that the parasite will be cleared without spreading. However, when R_0 is greater than 1, the pathogen will be passed on to at least one individual and it can spread within a population at a determined rate until control measures are taken to slow or stop this spread.

The basic reproductive ratio is also used to understand the possibility of an epidemic or pandemic taking place in emerging infectious disease. It has been used to understand the risk posed by the outbreak of SARS, bovine spongiform encephalitis (BSE or Creutzfeldt-Jakob Disease or 'mad cow' disease), foot and mouth disease, new strains of influenza, malaria, Ebola, and West Nile virus.

The same concept is used in the study of bioterrorism, indoor airborne infection, and also in the transmission of computer viruses.

There will be a number of factors that influence the spreadability of a pathogen. For example, if the onset of symptoms takes several days, and the pathogen is already infectious between its contraction and the symptoms appearing, this increases the chance of infecting other individuals before the infected person knows they are ill. This is called the incubation period. The series interval is also a determining factor. This is the time between the onset of symptoms in primary and secondary cases. Thus reproductive ration, serial interval, and incubation period all play a role in how fast the infection spreads within a population and can analyse whether there is a risk of epidemic or pandemic proportions.

HOW DOES COVID-19 MAKE YOU ILL?

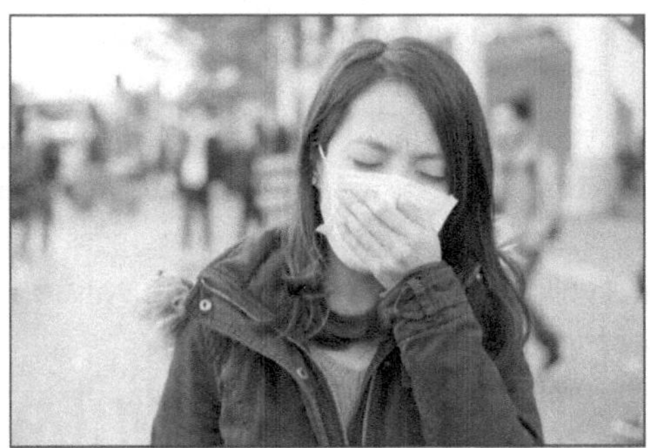

There are two ways to potentially contract the virus - from the faecal-oral route or through the respiratory droplet.

There have been several case studies that found the live infectious virus or viral RNA in faeces of patients, suggesting there may be a possibility of faecal-oral transmission. This means that particles may travel on the unwashed hands or fingernails of those infected after passing a stool. Viral particles may also be present on surfaces in the bathroom. This might also explain gastrointestinal symptoms such as nausea and vomiting or diarrhoea in some patients. Asymptomatic adults and children could be spreading the virus this way.

Airborne respiratory droplets released through coughing and sneezing can reach up to 2 metres or 6 feet. These droplets could also stay on surfaces for several hours, depending on the material in question. Particles with the virus may be airborne for potentially 3 hours so someone passing through the area could also get infected.

Once the virus enters the respiratory system through the lungs, it attacks the alveoli. These are tiny sacs through which the body conducts oxygen exchange with the atmosphere. Once the virus establishes itself within the alveoli, it attaches to type 2 pneumocytes. The role of these type 2 pneumocytes is normally to produce surfactant, which decreases the surface tension and reduces collapsing pressure of the alveoli. Type 1 pneumocytes also in the alveoli are for gas exchange.

The S-spike on the SARS-CoV-2 binds to specific receptors called angiotensin-converting enzyme Type 2 (ACE-2) on the type 2 pneumocyte cells. This allows for the virus to enter the cell, where it releases its positive-sense single-stranded RNA ((+)ssRNA). Once this is released, it can use the host cell's ribosomes, and via a process called translation, it converts the single-stranded RNA into specific protein molecules (polyproteins). The (+)ssRNA can also use another enzyme called the RNA-dependant RNA polymerase, which takes RNA and synthesises more RNA copies.

The polyproteins need to be used to make all the components of the viral structure, so different enzymes called proteinases are used to make these. These components - nucleocapsids, spike proteins, enzymes - are combined with the synthesised RNA to bud off from the host cell. Several viral structures have been manufactured inside the type 2 pneumocyte cells in the lungs of this patient.

In the process of the viral structures being released, this type 2 pneumocyte cell is destroyed with the result of releasing specific inflammatory mediators which attract and stimulate macrophages. Macrophages are cells whose purpose is to detect and remove cells it considers pathogens, as part of the immune system of the body. The macrophage which releases specific cytokines interleukin-1 (IL-1), inter-leukin-6 (IL-6), and tumor necrosis factor-alpha (TNF-α). These inflammatory mediators enter the bloodstream via the alveolar wall and cause the smooth muscle just outside the lungs to dilate. The endothelial cells in the muscle contract and this increases capillary permeability. These inflammatory mediators thus cause a number of events that lead plasma to leak into the interstitial spaces outside the alveoli. Some of the fluid enters the alveoli and causes oedema, leading to alveolar collapse. This decreases gas exchange via the type 1 pneumocytes. At this point, there is hypoxemia (low pressure of oxygen in the blood) and breathing becomes difficult because the surface area of the lungs has been compromised. This can present with increased work of breathing and shortness of breath and may lead to bilateral pneumonia.

The immune system of the body will also kick in due to these inflammatory mediators, and this will attract neutrophils which attack cells indiscriminately to destroy the virus. This helps to destroy more cells, even healthy ones, with the release of reactive oxygen species and proteases. As these different cells, including the virus, are destroyed and are released into the alveoli as debris. This further decreases the surface available for gas exchange. All of this cell debris and mucus containing sloughed cells and viral particles can then cause a cough, with the release of the virus into the air and possibly infection of a new host.

When IL-1, IL-6, and TNF-α are released in high concentrations, these can travel to the hypothalamus in the brain. This is the part of the brain that controls temperature. Here specific prostaglandins are released, which alters the body's thermostat and causes fever. The sympathetic nervous system will also cause an increased heart rate in the infected patient. The inflammation in the lungs can get so severe that it can lead to acute respiratory distress, and eventually to septicaemia as the rest of the body is involved via the entire circulatory system. This can lead to multi-system organ failure.

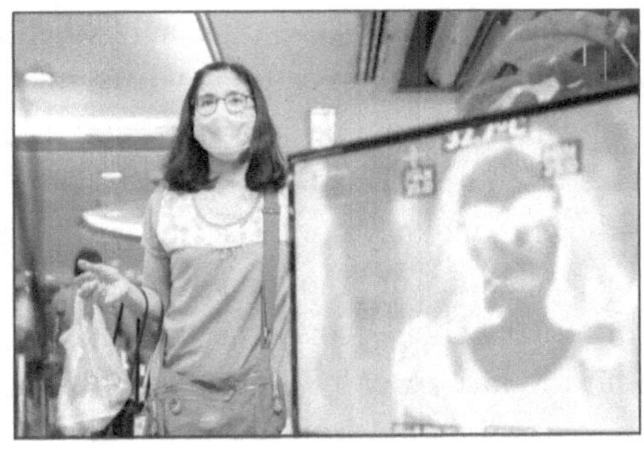

R_0 is a measure taken presuming normal circumstances. To decrease the degree of spreadability R_0 there are a number of non-pharmaceutical measures that can be taken. If there was prophylaxis (preventative medicine) or a cure for COVID-19 available at the start of the spread, these would be measures taken to decrease the spread too. However, with an infectious disease spreading fast, the only things we can do at first are non-pharmaceutical actions. The number of new cases of infection will directly depend on how efficiently these are conducted and the timing at which they are done.

As with any contagious disease, it is for the care of the community, to avoid spreading disease, that anyone exhibiting symptoms should stay at home until they are better. Crowded events, especially those held indoors, but also outdoor ones, are considered places of high risk. These should be avoided in the presence of a contagious pathogen in society.

Hygiene practices should be encouraged. This includes the frequent and thorough washing of hands with soap and water for 20-30 seconds. Using an alcohol rub between 60-80% alcohol is suggested if hand washing is not possible, especially when people are out of the home or in settings where infection is more likely. Nails should be kept short and using artificial nails discouraged, as these could harbour infectious pathogens and may not be cleaned as thoroughly.

When coughing or sneezing, the crook of the elbow or a tissue should cover the mouth. The patient should turn to face away from other people if possible. Any tissue used should be discarded safely immediately after use.

Since the virus is spread via droplets, it is important to avoid touching the face and therefore the respiratory airways and mucous membranes through which the virus may enter the respiratory tract. The virus may remain viable on a number of surfaces for a varying amount of time. So, for example, one may avoid getting the virus on the hands by turning switches on/off with the elbow instead of the hands. This avoids contact with the hands which are more likely to spread the virus to the face. Door handles, elevator buttons, handrails, shop counters, and cash are other materials that can present a frequent possibility of exposure, especially if these are in public places of high traffic. High awareness of what is being touched is important to recognise the frequency of hand-washing or disinfection with alcohol rub needed.

Social distance entails interacting with everyone at a distance which is larger than what we are used to. For example, when queuing in line, distances of 1-2 metres should be respected. In small shops, patrons should only be allowed to enter one or two at a time and sometimes not enter the shop at all, making the order from the outside of the shop. Social distancing also means we keep the interactions with people we don't live with to a minimum. The general population should keep outdoor interactions to a minimum, only going out for errands or activities (exercise, walking dogs) that are considered essential in their daily routine.

To this end, governments in most countries rolled out and enforced regulations to close services deemed to be non-essential, e.g., retail outlets, beauty parlours, restaurants. Most of these were allowed to offer their service in a different way. Restaurants could offer take-out or delivery services and retail outlets could offer online shopping. Work practices and delivery methods had to be changed to keep everyone safer, with increased safety and hygiene measures within and outside of such outlets. Payment using online methods is encouraged to avoid using cash, and having cash exchange hands. Deliveries are conducted in a 'contactless' manner whereby packages including food are left behind doors, with the delivery person distancing themselves while the package is collected.

Personal protective equipment (PPE) was and has been a frequently discussed topic as the pandemic situation with covid-19 unfolded. PPE includes face masks that cover the nose and mouth, gloves, goggles or other face shields that cover either the eyes only or most of the face, hair shields, and complete suits called 'hazmats' meaning hazardous material protection.

While using PPE is definitely warranted in health-care settings, it must be highlighted that without the knowledge of correct use, certain PPE may actually pose risks rather than protection. Masks and gloves must be applied and removed correctly in order not to touch the contaminated sides. People wearing gloves must be made aware these have the potential to harbour the virus and spread it to other surfaces that are touched. When used with sick patients, healthcare professionals should change gloves after each patient. In other circumstances, it is debatable whether using gloves is suggested, but it may be a good way to avoid touching the face.

The Centers for Disease Control and Prevention (CDC) was initially recommending the use of masks only when working in conditions considered of high risk (e.g., clinics and hospitals), and for patients who are ill. As of the 4th of April 2020, the CDC recommended that face coverings should be worn in public especially where social distancing measures may be difficult to uphold (e.g., grocery stores). Due to the lack of availability of masks considered appropriate for protecting the wearer from the virus entering, most

masks will instead decrease the output of virus particles if the wearer is a carrier of the virus (whether they
have symptoms or not). Even though this is not the
most ideal situation, it is offering a measure of protection considered better than not wearing any face
covering. Here, the danger which applies to wearing
gloves also applies. According to the CDC, cloth
coverings should fit snugly against the face without
restricting the airways; they should be secured with
ties or ear loops; they should preferably have multiple
layers of fabric. This is considered a voluntary public
health measure - a measure also enforced during the
1918 pandemic.

Frequently touched surfaces should be cleaned and
disinfected daily, and more often in households with
people who are ill or have tested positive for COVID-
19 (or other contagious illness). As much as possible,
those who are ill should stay in a specific room and
away from other people in the home. If a separate
bathroom is not available, this should be cleaned and
disinfected after being used by the person who is ill.
Gloves should be worn during the cleaning and
discarded after each cleaning. If the gloves used are
not disposable, these should be kept for this sole
purpose. When surfaces are dirty, these should be
cleaned with regular soap prior to disinfection.

The general public has also been advised to practice hygiene with objects brought into the home from
the outside. Shoes should be left outside of the house
or in designated areas, the soles disinfected so as not
to introduce any contamination into the rest of the
home. Groceries should either be wiped down or not
touched for a few days, giving the possible viral load

time to decrease. It is thought that the virus can remain viable for around 24 hours on paper and cardboard, 4 hours on copper, and up to 72 hours on stainless steel surfaces. It can also linger in the air for up to 3 hours, for example, if someone has been sneezing in a room with poor ventilation.

WHO IS MOST PRONE?

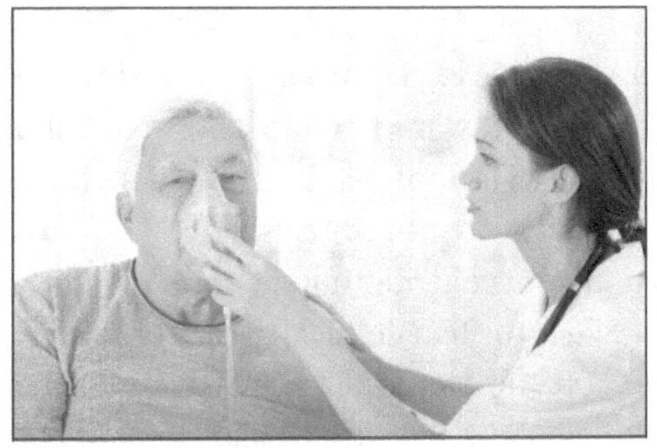

For some people, an infection with COVID-19 may pose a higher risk of complications. Those considered more vulnerable are older people (65 years and up) and people of any age suffering from a number of underlying medical conditions. Patients with compromised immunity, such as those who are HIV+ or have poorly controlled AIDS , those receiving cancer treatment, those who have had bone marrow or organ transplantation, or who have been under corticosteroid care are more at risk of developing severe complications once they get infected. Other risk factors include cardiovascular disease, severe obesity, diabetes, moderate to severe asthma, and chronic kidney or liver disease.

Death with COVID-19 has been observed mostly in males of over 70 with concurrent comorbidities such as respiratory disease or cardiovascular disease. It is yet unknown why the disease has killed more males, but it is thought that it may be connected to the fact that males were more likely to be smokers and, therefore, also have subsequent related comorbidities. Obesity was also highly associated with these increased risks. Both smoking and obesity were observed as big, contributing factors to the high number of deaths experienced in Italy. However, when comparing deaths in Italy to those in China, and perhaps due to lack of details in the data from China, these findings were not conclusive.

Two other contributing factors for the rate of higher male to female deaths are a difference in hygiene and the fact that males have higher rates of preexisting conditions such as diabetes and high blood pressure. These factors make those who contract the disease more vulnerable to severe complications that may lead to death. This trend was in patients from China, Italy, France, Germany, Iran, and South Korea. According to the Italian National Health Service, as of March 20th, 2020, approximately 70% of deaths in Italy were male, even though there was only a slight male majority of those infected. It is estimated that around 7 million males smoke in Italy, compared to 4.5 million women. Smokers have a higher risk of requiring ventilation and intensive care once they contract COVID-19.

Unlike some other viruses, SARS-CoV-2 rarely causes infection in babies and children, and even when an infection is symptomatic, there is a very low risk of severe disease.

PANDEMIC PREPAREDNESS

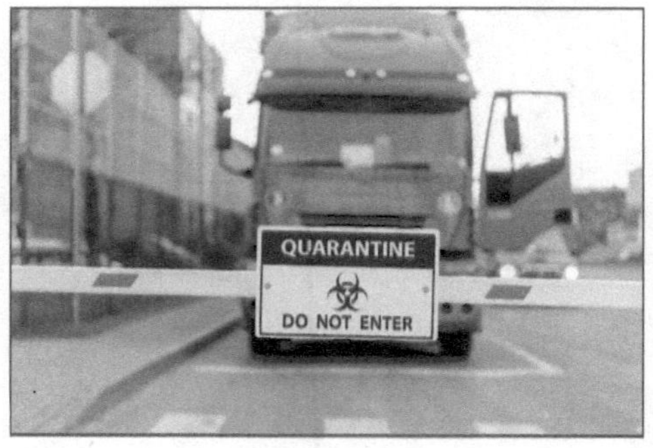

The term 'preparedness' describes how healthcare systems, governments, professional response organisations, businesses, communities, and individuals can respond or react effectively to the emergence and establishment of a particular event. Usually, we use 'preparedness' for something that is likely to happen or that we expect to happen imminently, by means of risk assessment.

Risk assessment analysis is an exercise conducted periodically to understand which hazardous events may happen. It is why for every entity from governments to private businesses to have such a contingency plan in place to protect its people and ensure business continuity occurs as much as possible. This may mean that a support system is in place that may not be used for a while or may never be used. It may be loosely compared to having a first aid box that holds sufficient and extensive materials to be of help to many people at once. It is also a system that needs to be assessed periodically to ensure that it is still up to date and that it can still function bearing in mind any new risk that may have arisen since the last assessment.

Keeping the same analogy of the first aid box - it is insufficient to have the materials at hand if people are not trained to apply CPR, use a bandage, or clean a wound. This training must be repeated every few years; new employees may need to be trained; the first aid materials may need to be replenished or replaced upon expiry.

By improving the speed and quality by which a response can be made, and by providing an infrastructure for the response, there can be a major difference in attaining the goal, be it of saving lives, reducing suffering, or achieving a more seamless business continuity.

Preparedness and continuity should be part of a business or government's standard operating procedures (SOPs). With the evolution of scientific knowledge and a knowledge of history, certain events can also be predicted. This is important in the design of preparedness.

With zoonotic viruses periodically hopping across the species barrier, and with some presenting as killers, especially when they are new, it was only a matter of time until another pandemic occurred.

The Spanish flu pandemic, which occurred in 1918, has been the worst flu pandemic on record to date. There have been several flu pandemics since, but these were milder ones. These pandemics have been caused by the influenza type A virus, with birds and some mammals being the reservoir for this. By studying the progress of previous pandemics, especially those in more recent history, experts can determine which measures have been more successful in curbing the spread of infection to minimise disease and deaths.

Although every virus and its resulting disease is different, the 1918 pandemic has often been taken as a model and its dynamics studied for preparedness. With globalisation and a growing population being just two of many factors that may increase the spread of an infectious disease quite quickly, it was envisioned that it would only be a matter of time until the next big pandemic hit the planet.

Despite having this knowledge, and despite the fact that some countries have had contingency plans in place for the next pandemic, it seems that no one was prepared enough for what COVID-19 brought about. One reason is that each virus will behave differently, and it may be challenging not only to judge which measures should be set into motion but also to decide on the timing of such measures.

Historically the most useful non-pharmaceutical measure to slow down the spread of infection has been social distancing. That is, the avoidance of the formation of groups or crowds of people. This is done by closing schools, places of worship, bars and restaurants, and other non-essential shops, outlets, and services. Another measure is to quarantine those who are ill and anyone who may have come in contact with them. Those people over 65 or with compromised immune systems are advised to stay at home as much as possible, and only come into contact with people they are living with.

These measures all aim at 'flattening the curve', that is making sure that the number of ill people does not rise suddenly and overwhelm the healthcare system. Instead, a gradual increase of cases over time is preferred, in that all patients will have better access to care without causing the healthcare system to work at full capacity and more.

When the healthcare system is pushed to full capacity, many factors limit the level of care that can be given. For example, during this particular pandemic, some of the more severe cases will need to be placed on ventilators. When there aren't sufficient ventilators, doctors need to choose which patients will be placed on the equipment, and others may risk losing their life. Another factor is these patients may need to be placed in buildings that were not designed to be hospitals, such as the temporary hospitals erected for a time in China when coronavirus hit them the worst.

Temporary hospitals need to be staffed and health systems may need to call in extra help in the form of retired healthcare professionals or healthcare students. Keeping patients in quarantine so as not to infect others would be an issue. And finally, a very important point to remember is this means that nurses, doctors, pharmacists, lab technicians, cleaners and all other hospital staff would be overworked, at risk of getting the infection or of taking the infection home to their family. Some of them have chosen to live away from their family while they are caring for the ill during this pandemic. They would also suffer from high levels of anxiety and stress due to these worries and from being exhausted.

Care homes, prisons, convents, and other places where several people live together are also places that might suffer in a particular way during a pandemic. Often nurses, carers, administrative staff, cleaners, and guards may need to go on lockdown inside these facilities to avoid the risk that people going in and out of the buildings may bring. This is especially important in care homes where the elderly are already in a vulnerable position and may suffer from comorbidities that would place them in further danger.

'Flattening the curve'

One phrase we've heard mentioned often during this pandemic is 'flattening the curve,' and the non-pharmaceutical actions and precautions suggested aim at achieving this. The term explains the best strategy available at the time to stop the COVID-19 spread. This curve represents the cases (infected people) on a given day versus time passing (in terms of days). Ideally, the number of total cases would be decreased, but here the focus is multifaceted and aims at spreading the cases over a longer period of time. In the representation, a line is drawn across the middle where the healthcare capacity is presumed to reach its peak. One curve is drawn with a fictional scenario in mind - that of not taking any protective measures against COVID-19. Another curve shows how the spread would be when enough protective measures are taken in a timely manner.

In the envisioned ideal spread (the curve where protective measures are taken) time is passing and therefore allowing the healthcare system to care for the ill, having recoveries and clearing out beds and any medical apparatus needed for the new cases. This interruption of the natural flow of the outbreak is essential for hospitals and their healthcare professionals to best deal with their patients.

Consider that a (yet unknown) percentage of cases would require hospital care, and all cases should ideally be in isolation from other people. An emphasis is placed on allowing the healthcare system enough time to cope with the number of cases rather than overwhelming it with a steep rise of infected patients. An exponential increase in cases such as that seen in Italy in the first few weeks of infections is exactly what experts are afraid of. Not having enough beds and space in hospital facilities, the need to build makeshift hospitals, and other patient treatment areas, and failing to catch up demand can quickly bring the healthcare system to its knees.

Professionals advise that the spread can be slowed down by practicing social distancing. This means that people avoid public spaces, limit their movements outside of the home, and leave space between themselves and other people. In many countries, people were soon asked to stay at home unless they needed to go out for something essential. Businesses were encouraged to let employees work from home if this was possible. Others limited their working hours and adopted new measures to ensure that their employees and customers could keep themselves safe. Some businesses that offered one to one services where social distancing is not possible, e.g., barbers, beauty salons, had to shut their doors, either voluntarily or following orders from their country's government. Restaurants and bars faced the same fate, as they are places where gathering in groups is encouraged. Small and large eateries had to change their business model to introduce take-out or delivery of food ranging from fast food to Michelin star food and everything in between. Services deemed non-essential, such as retail outlets and malls, were asked to close. Large local and international events such as concerts and conferences were postponed, canceled, or taken to online platforms.

The timing adopted by different countries depended on decisions taken by their experts, but also decisions taken by their leaders and politicians, and these weren't always on the same page. Aside from that, measures taken sometimes depended on the cooperation of the general public, and this varied depending on the culture of the country and the kind of socialising they were prone to do. The strictness of the measures also made a difference in that 'encouragement' was not 'enforcement', and 'enforcement' had a varying degree of consequence.

Flattening the curve to spread out the cases also gives scientists and researchers more time to learn about the virus and its behaviour. Buying some weeks during which the cases are decreased may mean limiting deaths to a certain degree until when we learn of a possible cure or confirm that a vaccine is effective and safe for use. Diagnostic tests can also be improved with time and gained knowledge. Devices needed in the care of critical patients, for example, ventilators, need to be increased in number in the most hard-hit countries. Other accessories for use during the pandemic, such as sanitizer gels and masks, also need to be obtained. All of this takes time, and although social distancing measures may be difficult for some, it is a measure that may prove successful if done right.

SOCIAL ISSUES OF SELF-ISOLATION

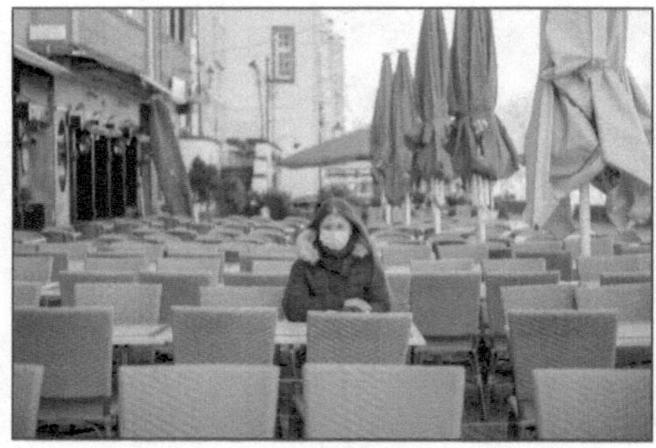

The way people live has a considerable influence on social distancing. Social issues intensify at times of global emergency, yet we scarcely have the time to consider them.

If your job is one where you can **work from home**, there are other complications around you to consider. Will your partner also be working from home? Do you own two computers or laptops? If you have children and the schools are shut, you may suddenly be in a position where you need to take care of them, perhaps offer them some homeschooling, or give up some of your time at the computer so they can watch their lessons. Will one parent need to give up their job or reduce their hours? Will it be possible to juggle all of these obligations, and what are the health implications of doing so? What happens to single parents with young children?

Migrants, who may already live in squalid conditions, and in close proximity with many others, are a particular risk group. They may not have access to information and may receive partial or incorrect messages on what to do during this time. The simple messages of washing hands often, not touching your face, self-isolating, especially when ill, stopping non-essential activities, and keeping a distance from other people who don't live with you, may not arrive to them. They may also be perceived badly by a person who has been treated as an outsider.

Those who have just managed to start establishing themselves in society may be reluctant to take these steps, that may seem counterintuitive in the narrative of their life. Those with a job have worked hard to get it and will be once again thrown into a situation where they cannot provide for themselves and their family. The dynamic with volunteers may be altered as this is a double-edged sword. Does one risk bringing the infection into a community living in close quarters? Is the information available so new behaviour is adopted?

In the UK, a large number of NGOs, organizations, and charities have teamed up to support vulnerable migrants during the COVID-19 pandemic by asking local authorities to take 'urgent steps' to protect them. The UN migration agency also highlighted the importance of treating migrants with respect and dignity, pointing out that many had been working in industries now shut down due to the current situation. They are demanding equal access to public health and pointed at the danger of ignoring this large part of society. The UN migration agency expressed the fear that COVID-19 is associated with being something foreign, something that comes from travellers, and this may cause further discrimination. They have and will be taking special measures to protect migrants during this time.

In late March 2020, Portugal declared that they will be treating migrants as permanent residents during the pandemic - which will mean access to the country's healthcare service and welfare system. Migrants will be allowed to open bank accounts and will have the same conditions for work and rental contracts as locals do.

#Stayathome may be one of the buzzwords during the pandemic, but how will the **homeless** be affected by the pandemic? Will more people be pushed to the streets as jobs are lost, and families are unable to make rent? How long will it take until those living paycheck-to-paycheck find themselves in such situations? To those who are already homeless, this balance does not need to tip. They are already there.

With more outlets being ordered to close and people being urged to only make essential trips, there is far less foot traffic in the streets. This means fewer opportunities for charity in the form of spare change or food. Without heated public spaces, and the availability of restrooms, how will the homeless cope?

There already aren't enough shelters for the homeless, and though voluntary groups try to take care of the homeless population, things may be about to get worse. Unsheltered people often live in unhygienic conditions with a lack of access to running water, making frequent hand washing impossible. They often suffer from respiratory diseases and other comorbidities. When they live in communities, they are often in close proximity to each other and may huddle in groups to keep warm. What happens if they become ill or carriers of the virus?

To begin tackling these worrying issues, a number of US states are calling for a temporary moratorium on evictions from homes as well as businesses to minimise the number of people becoming newly homeless. Landlords in these states are under obligation to comply with this or face fees. In some countries, landlords have taken this decision of their own accord and have temporarily lowered or completely eliminated rent due. They have done this to safeguard those renting their properties who may be going through a difficult time due to lay-offs, temporary closures, or forced quarantine due to exposure to COVID-19 or illness with it.

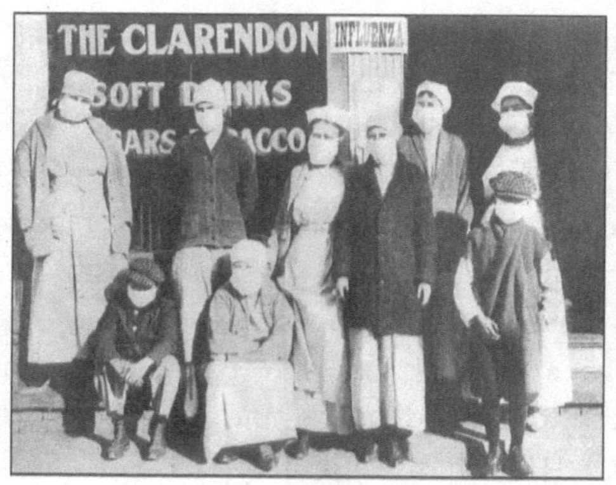

The 1918 Spanish flu was caused by an H1N1 influenza virus over 100 years ago. It is estimated that 50 million people worldwide died during that pandemic, and this death rate had not been observed during any flu season before, nor has it been observed since. The curious characteristic of this virus was that it caused a high death rate among healthy, young adults.

This deadly virus could hold useful hints for

researchers as they try to uncover why it was so deadly and where it came from. Unravelling this event in history could hold the key to understanding many properties of viral infection in the fight against the current and future pandemics.

How does the Spanish flu compare to COVID-19? Both infections affect the respiratory system and can lead to pneumonia. In COVID-19, one of the more common symptoms is shortness of breath, often accompanied by fever and a cough, which is generally dry. However, the two viruses belong to different families and are not traced back to the same origins or hosts. As the new coronavirus makes its way around the world, experts have been turning to the deadliest pandemic in modern history to examine the best options for dealing with a global pandemic.

Despite the difference in what they knew then and what we know now, the efforts implemented then to stem the spread may offer lessons for today. A large difference can be observed between US cities in their non-pharmaceutical measures taken when they were taken and to what extent, and the number of deaths they suffered.

In Philadelphia, the death rate was high because they waited eight days after deaths began to ban social gatherings and close schools. They experienced the highest peak death rate of the cities studied. The city also hosted a parade attended by 200,000 people 10 days after this first death. On the other hand, St. Louis had strong social distancing measures in place. The city delayed the peak in deaths and also had a low total death rate. However, when the regulations were temporarily eased, there was a sharp increase in the culmination of deaths.

Another marked difference between the Spanish flu and COVID-19 is the age group considered most vulnerable to infection. In the Spanish flu pandemic, there was unusually high mortality in young adults; thus, it—was affecting people who were generally healthy. COVID-19 is most dangerous to those with weak immune systems, such as older people and those with comorbidities such as heart problems, diabetes, respiratory illness and others. Although this has generally been the norm, some adults deemed to be generally healthy have suffered greatly and even died from COVID-19. Younger adults, adolescents, and children may exhibit milder symptoms and sometimes no symptoms at all, even when they test positive.

We can get a sense of the overall trajectory of COVID-19 compared to the Spanish flu because we have a hint of its reproductive rate. Although it is early to know exactly how fast COVID-19 infection is spreading, and since some people remain asymptomatic, we do know that it is more easily transmittable than the yearly flu, putting the reproductive rate between 2-2.5. It is estimated that the Spanish flu had a reproductive rate of around 1.8. It is estimated that between 20-60% of the population will eventually become infected with the novel coronavirus.

It is the stealth by which COVID-19 is transmitted often under the radar, with mild or no symptoms, that makes it all the more dangerous, and makes the need for social distancing even more important. If the method of testing in a particular country is not proactively looking for cases, but only testing those with symptoms and tracing their immediate contacts, there is no way of really knowing just how far the infection has spread and who poses a danger to others by being an asymptomatic carrier.

The spread of COVID-19 has been swift due to globalisation. The first spread out of Wuhan, China, and into Europe and America was via air travel, a means nowadays accessible to many. This could happen very fast as opposed to travel in 1918, which happened via rail and sea. Historians believe that the Spanish flu spread was tied to troops being sent to fight in World War I.

With the Spanish flu, the fatality rate was thought to be between 10-20 percent. At present, the fatality rate of COVID-19 seems much lower, but it has varied significantly between countries. This depends on a number of factors, such as if the country has an aging population, how many tests are conducted, and what kind of social distancing practices have been put into place or enforced. As of the end of March, the general mortality rate was around 4.8% when taking the worldwide total confirmed cases and an official count of the total deceased patients.

As of the end of March, we are still living in what will probably be considered the 'first wave' of the coronavirus pandemic. The Spanish flu lasted for 2 years in all, but the worst period of time was the end of the year 1918 when the majority of deaths occurred. The world population is much larger now than it was in 1918 when 500 million people contracted the disease - this was one-third of the world's population. The number of deaths at the time was estimated to be up to 50 million. In the second wave of the Spanish flu pandemic, a surge in cases was caused by a mutation of the virus, and again this was thought to have been caused by the flow by wartime troops.

Since the 1918 pandemic occurred during wartime, efforts and finances were mostly diverted towards war efforts, and the public health system was not a priority. Besides that, it was only the middle class and wealthy who could afford access to healthcare. Those who lived in poorer conditions, especially in areas lacking good hygiene, suffered and died in greater numbers. Even though healthcare systems in developing countries may be weak, there is an availability of healthcare professionals and hospitals to look after patients. In most countries, even the impoverished citizens can get some medical attention.

With medical innovations made in the last 100+ years, scientists and health experts around the world are armed with resources and knowledge to test new options for prophylaxis, protocols, cures, and a vaccine in the fight against the new coronavirus. Examining the behaviour of previous pandemics and epidemics, as well as studying patterns of what worked to curb the spread and what didn't, is crucial in learning the best way forward in containing this new threat.

SARS

The outbreak of Severe Acute Respiratory Syndrome (SARS) caused by what was later named SARS-CoV (SARS Coronavirus) started in 2002 via a coronavirus very similar in structure to SARS-CoV-2. That was the first introduction of a coronavirus, which caused severe symptoms in the human population in the twenty-first century. Before that, the known coronaviruses, which were pathogenic to humans, caused mild respiratory symptoms and did not cause alarm. Thus the need to investigate this type of virus further was not a priority until SARS-CoV came along.

SARS was caused by a previously unknown (therefore 'new' or 'novel') animal coronavirus that mutated to be contagious and infectious in humans. It is thought that this virus exploited the setting provided by 'wet markets' in southern China to affect the spillover into humans. It also adapted or mutated in such a way that human to human transmission became possible. The first few patients were all related to the wet market in Guangdong province. In certain regions, such as Guangdong province, the demand for 'exotic' animals has increased with increased affluence. Thus, such markets have increased in number and size to be able to cater for increased trade in restaurants and their demand for such live 'wild' animal species.

When blood samples were taken from healthy workers that had dealt with animals in these wet markets, antibodies that matched those to SARS-CoV virus were found, even though these people had not had SARS-like illness. This may indicate that earlier transmission was weak and may have only caused minor symptoms or none at all. It also indicated that at an earlier stage, the human-to-human transmission was not effective. Eventually, the virus adapted to more efficient human-to-human disease, and this set off the cascade of events that led to the pandemic.

Specimens were also collected from seemingly healthy animals, including Himalayan palm civets, found in the live-game markets in Guangdong also resulted in a SARS-CoV-like virus which matched the nucleotide homology of the human SARS-CoV by

99%. Bats are thought to be the natural reservoirs for SARS-like coronaviruses. Following several studies, it was found that SARS-CoV-like viruses that matched the nucleotide homology of the human SARS-CoV shared 88-92% similarity with those detected in a species of Chinese horseshoe bats. This bat exists in the wild in Hong Kong and Southern China.

An examination of palm civets raised in a farm used to supply the wet market resulted in an absence of these antibodies against SARS-CoV-like viruses, implying these animals were not the natural reservoir of the virus but that they contracted the virus in the market (probably via horseshoe bats) and perpetuated it there.

Clusters of disease appeared in families and in healthcare workers that had treated patients with this 'infectious atypical pneumonia'. At the time travellers and hospitals augmented the spread that permitted it to become an outbreak of global proportions.

One such example is the physician from Guang-dong Province in China who stayed in the hotel 'M' in Hong Kong on February 21st, 2003. During this day, he transmitted the infection to 16 other guests who passed on the infection to others in Hong Kong, Singapore, Vietnam, and Toronto. An outbreak resulted in each of these places, and within weeks the SARS infection had affected more than 8000 people in 25 countries across 5 continents.

SARS-CoV is an airborne virus, and it is transmitted in a similar way to colds and the flu, which is via small droplets in saliva when an infected person coughs or sneezes into the air and that air is breathed in. It can also be spread indirectly via surfaces such as when an infected person touches door handles, stair rails, and lift buttons. A healthy person may then touch these within a short space of time, and then touch their face, in particular mucous membranes such as the nose, mouth, and eyes. The virus may then enter the body via these mucous membranes and may establish infection in the airways.

Symptoms of SARS illness are similar to those that occur with the flu and begin 2-7 days following infection. Sometimes the incubation period after coming into contact with the virus can be up to 10 days. These symptoms include fever, chills, muscle pain, extreme tiredness, headaches, loss of appetite, and diarrhoea. Following these symptoms, the infection affects the lower respiratory system to cause a dry cough, a lower level of oxygen in the blood, and breathing difficulties. These symptoms have the potential to be fatal in severe cases.

The pandemic was brought under control in July 2003 when patients with suspected SARS were kept isolated, and all passengers travelling by air from and within affected areas were screened for infection.

A second outbreak happened in 2004, which was identified back to someone coming into direct contact with a sample of SARS virus in a medical lab in China. Therefore, in this case, there was no animal-to-human contact or human-to-human contagion. There have been no other reported cases of SARS since 2004 to date.

During the infection period, SARS had a mortality rate of 10%. There were a total of 774 deaths and 8098 reported cases of illness with SARS.

The global response of isolating all infected patients as soon as possible after symptoms showed up succeeded in decreasing and finally eliminating further transmission. Several years have passed without the re-emergence of SARS in humans, though the potential for re-introduction from animals to humans via a natural animal reservoir or spillage from a research lab still exists. This highlights the need to be hypervigilant when atypical or severe respiratory symptoms appear. Stringent practices should be in place to react in a timely manner on such occasions before hospital transmission, or transmission among family units can occur.

MERS

Middle East Respiratory Syndrome coronavirus (MERS-CoV) first appeared in 2012 as a new viral pathogen affecting humans. All MERS cases were linked directly or indirectly to the Middle East region but have been reported in the later phases in other countries within Europe.

The average incubation period of this virus was reported to be 5.2 days, slightly longer than with SARS-CoV. The case fatality was higher with MERS-CoV, reaching around 30%. MERS has also been reported to cause a greater disruption to the body's immune response. The fatality rate may be misleading since it is hard to know how many people were infected without showing any symptoms or showing only very mild symptoms that may have been mistaken for another infection without being tested.

This marked the second emergence of a highly infectious coronavirus into the human population during the 21st century. It is thought that MERS-CoV was introduced into the human population via dromedary camels following cross-species transmission from bats, the reservoir animal of this coronavirus. Even though bats are the reservoir animal, it is unlikely that most patients who got ill came into contact with infected bats, since this kind of interaction is uncommon. The zoonotic transmission between dromedary camels and humans is described as continuous, which means that unprotected contact with dromedary camels still poses a risk.

The first case was reported in June 2012 in Jeddah, Saudi Arabia. This was a decade after the outbreak with SARS-CoV in 2002. MERS exhibited an inefficient spread between humans, suggesting that zoonotic transmission was responsible for this infection. Genetic sequencing has revealed the presence of CoV RNA in the fecal samples of bats in Africa, Asia, and Europe, some of which closely resemble MERS-CoV. Evidence has also been found in dromedary camels, which had high levels of antibodies, infectious viruses, and viral RNA, suggesting a past infection with MERS-CoV or a closely-related virus. Unpasteurized camel milk was also found to contain the virus and could be another source of infection. Cautions against consuming unpasteurized milk and having close association with dromedary camels were issued by the WHO, Saudi Arabia, and Qatar.

MERS-CoV results in acute pneumonia which is highly fatal, and renal dysfunction either due to damage from deprivation of oxygen or direct infection of the kidney. The symptoms seen include fever, cough, difficulty breathing, sore throat, chest pain, myalgia, and gastrointestinal issues such as abdominal pain, vomiting, or diarrhoea. During early infection, the virus can only be detected in the upper respiratory tract, while in the later stages, it can be detected in the lower respiratory tract. The fact that in some cases it has been detected in the blood and urine of patients indicates there is possibly systemic infection too.

Vulnerable and immunocompromised patients are at a higher risk of suffering from major complications following infection with MERS-CoV. The most at risk were those suffering from obesity, diabetes mellitus, asthma, cystic fibrosis, end-stage renal disease, cardiac disease, hypertension, and other immunosuppressive conditions. In cases of MERS infection, secondary infection with another agent was also reported frequently.

Unlike SARS, which was completely eliminated from the human population within 2 years, MERS cases continue to appear until 2020. To this day, 80% of cases continue to be reported by Saudi Arabia, with people getting infected through infected people or via unprotected contact with dromedary camels. Travelers who get infected have usually been to the Middle East. Virus transmission has occurred in healthcare facilities in several countries. This includes transmission between patients and from patients to healthcare providers. It is sometimes difficult to recognise the symptoms of MERS, especially if they are non-specific or mild. Healthcare providers should be made aware and trained appropriately in the prevention and control of infection. Such measures should be in place to prevent the possible spread of MERS within these facilities, especially in the more prone areas.

Safety measures should be in place so anyone visiting a farm or any place where dromedary camels are present should practice hygiene measures, such as hand washing before and after touching the animals. Contact with sick animals should be avoided. Animal products, including camel meat and camel milk, are deemed safe if they are processed properly - meat should be cooked thoroughly and milk pasteurized. All animal products should be handled with care to avoid cross-contamination with uncooked products.

Lessons learned from SARS and MERS threats

After both SARS and MERS threats, experts highlighted the need for a better understanding of the establishment of infection and the need for a system of control measures in case of new threats. The potential for a new coronavirus to appear in humans via zoonosis is always present since these viruses continue to spill over from the animal kingdom. This is more likely where interaction with animals and their habitats is more pronounced, where humans encroach on areas previously inhabited by animals, and where animals are kept in unnatural circumstances, such as in cages and in wet markets.

Researchers also highlighted the importance of isolating viral proteins, which are most involved in infection to develop models on which to study pathogenesis further.

UNHEEDED WARNINGS FROM EXPERTS

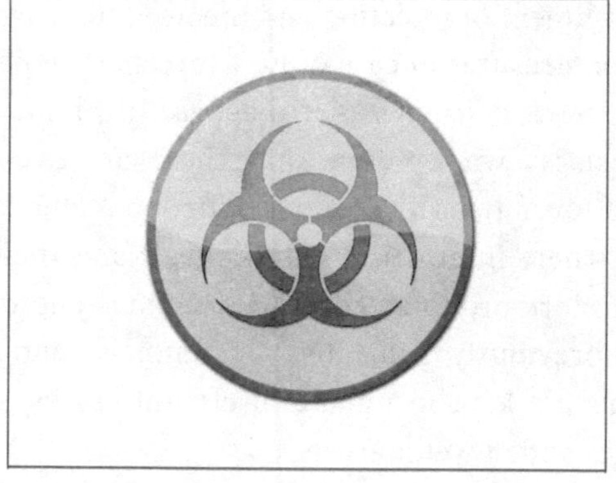

In September 2019, merely months before the first cases of COVID-19 were made official by China, the Global Preparedness Monitoring Board (GPMB) released a report titled 'A World At Risk'. This was an annual report on global preparedness for health emergencies. The GPMB is an independent body that urges and supports political action in the preparedness and mitigation of the impact of global health emergencies. This assembly was brought together by the World

Bank Group and the World Health Organization (WHO), and it built on the work of the Global Health Crises Task Force and Panel, initiated following the 2014-2016 Ebola epidemic.

The aims of the Board were to understand the world's capability for protection during health emergencies, identify gaps in this preparedness to mitigate such crises from various angles, and urge decision-makers and leaders to put in place measures for preparedness. They were focusing in particular on risks of a biological nature that would cause epidemics and pandemics. Because of this, they would be pushing for particular actions to effect change, considering those inconsistencies revealed by recent outbreaks.

The GPMB considered the particular problem of a fast-moving virulent respiratory pathogen that might be introduced into society via natural or artificial means, with a concern that the world is not prepared for such an event. The United Nations and WHO describe preparedness as 'the ability (knowledge, capacities, and organizational systems) of governments, professional response organizations, communities and individuals to anticipate, detect and respond effectively to, and recover from, the impact of likely, imminent or current health emergencies, hazards, events or conditions. It means putting in place mechanisms that will allow national authorities, multilateral organizations and relief organizations to be aware of risks and deploy staff and resources quickly once a crisis strikes.'

The GPMB called for 7 urgent actions to take place to prepare the world for health emergencies:

. . .

1. Heads of government must commit to the International Health Regulations (IHR) set in 2005. They should invest in repeated spending for preparedness. Continuous community engagement should be in place for detecting outbreaks early, controlling the spread, ensuring trust, and promoting effective responses. Each national leader should recognise their obligation not just to their country but to the world. The IHR agreement binds governments to foster readiness in their country in terms of the ability to detect, investigate, report, and counteract health threats. They should also have a reporting system to alter the WHO of such matters in a timely manner.

2. Countries and regional organizations should lead by example by going ahead with funding commitments for preparedness. They should also routinely assess progress during their annual meetings.

3. Each country should have a strong system in place with an independent high-level coordinator having jurisdiction and liability.

4. The level of preparedness by countries, donors, and global institutions must be for the worst-case scenario. An emphasis was placed on being prepared for a virulent lethal respiratory pathogen that would cause a rapidly-spreading pandemic. Therefore the report highlighted the need for tools and systems to respond effectively to such a scenario: to put in place non-pharmaceutical measures, identify and sequence a new pathogen, share information with the rest of the world, and finally to create therapeutics, prophylaxis, or a vaccine. The shared manufacturing of vaccines should ideally begin days after the sequencing of the pathogen has been done and shared with the rest of the world. With effective preparedness, the goal is to

have a vaccine in place approved for use within weeks of the discovery and sequencing of a new pathogen.

5. Financial institutions must link preparedness with financial risk planning.

6. Development assistance funders should create incentives and increase funding for preparedness. Those countries considered poor or more vulnerable should get increased funding and greater or earlier access to the United Nations Central Emergency Response Fund.

7. The United Nations must bolster coordination mechanisms for a comprehensive response to health threats and emergencies in different countries and under different health and emergency contexts.

The GPMB recognised shortcomings during this exercise and made it clear that although response mechanisms have improved, as exhibited by the timeliness in detection and response to Ebola in 2018, the mechanisms in place were not sufficient to deal with the enormous impact of a highly lethal pandemic. They stated there are insufficient research and development investment and a subpar infrastructure to create vaccines and formulate new targeted therapies. The system for sharing the sequencing of new pathogens was also deemed inefficient, as were the means for the distribution of limited medical resources across countries.

If we compared with the losses suffered during the Spanish flu pandemic, considering a population that has grown by four times, and the ease by which most people can travel the world, it is possible that between 50-80 million people could die during a similar pandemic. In economic measures, the GPMB declared that epidemic or pandemic control costs would overwhelm the global economy, with a view that the increasingly globalised world is only as strong as its weakest link.

Preparedness is hampered by the fact that national leaders tend to respond to health crises only when there is an immediate need, and they do not devote consistent attention, financials, or resources to keep any outbreaks from escalating. Two-thirds of countries do not yet have the capacity required under IHR 2005. Low- and middle-income countries still cannot cope with the financial burden required to maintain these systems for preparedness.

Just months before the world was hit by the COVID-19 pandemic, experts warned governments about the extent of lack of pandemic preparedness we could be facing.

WHAT ARE WE FEELING DURING SELF-ISOLATION?

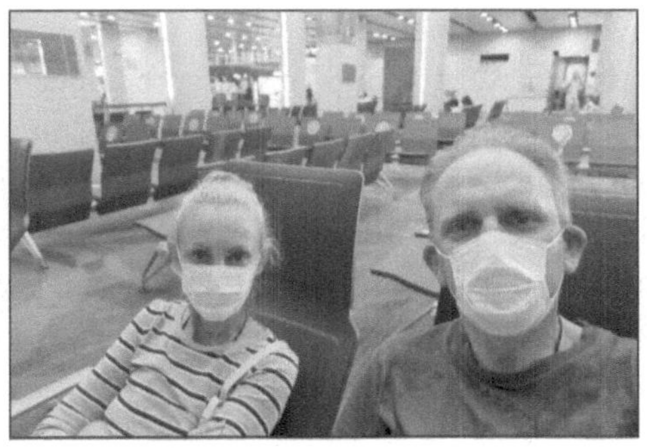

The discomfort we're feeling as COVID-19 changes life as we know it is a multi-faceted monster. David Kessler, a grief expert, shared his thoughts about how what we might be feeling is akin to grief. Acknowledging and giving a name to these feelings may be a big important step in understanding what we are going through.

Grief has a number of stages, and they don't necessarily present in a linear manner. There are also a number of different griefs. Understanding the stages of grief is a good way to be aware of what we are going through. These are denial, anger, bargaining, sadness, and acceptance.

Though we may be worried about death in general, death of a vulnerable loved one, or our own death, we are also grieving life as we know it. We have lost what we considered normal, lost the regular connections we had to the outside world and people we know lost our freedom to decide where to go and when. We have had to make do with new routines, with unplanned work from home that may be subpar. A contingency plan may have come at us faster than anticipated. We have lost a sense of future and aren't sure what to expect. We don't know if this storm will end, when it will end, and how we will emerge out of it.

Control may be found in the acceptance stage of this process, and it is where the strength to foster a community feel also lies. It is a time where you might be doing things or not doing things, not only because they affect you but also for the good and safety of others. This is when building a strong sense of compassion is vital.

FUTURE OUTLOOK - WHEN WILL WE HAVE A VACCINE AGAINST COVID-19?

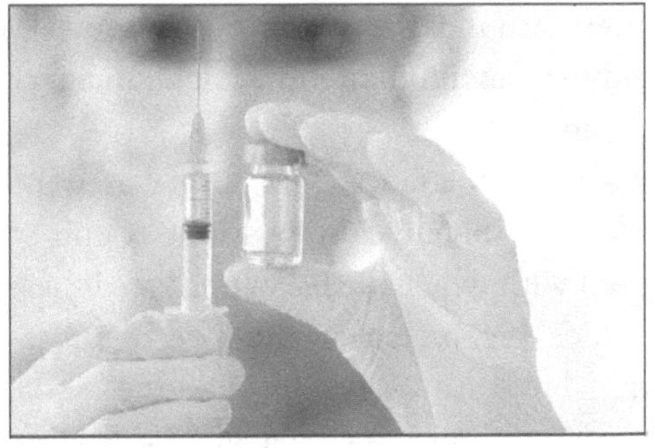

In mid-March Moderna Therapeutics, the developer of the first vaccine against COVID-19 to be tested administered the vaccine to their first set of volunteers. Testing of the vaccine may take almost a year, presuming this is found to be successful, but meanwhile, this work could provide valuable information on how the immune system can fight off coronaviruses. This is important to prepare researchers for any new emerging coronaviruses. Even if the frantic efforts of scientists to produce a vaccine doesn't pay off for some time, their work would not have been wasted.

About 35 companies and academic institutions have taken on the task of trying to create such a vaccine that can prevent people from developing COVID-19 now and in the future. While Moderna Therapeutics has started human trials, a few others have been testing on animals. Experts from all over the world have joined forces and offered their expertise in this concerted effort. Developing a vaccine could be started so soon after the onset of this pandemic thanks to the efforts of Chinese experts who sequenced the genetic material of SARS-CoV-2 in early January 2020. Through sharing this genetic coding, researchers around the world could grow the virus and study its method in invading human cells and making people ill.

Richard Hatchett, CEO of Oslo-based nonprofit Coalition for Epidemic Innovations (Cepi) said that 'The speed with which we have [produced these candidates] builds very much on the investment in understanding how to develop vaccines for other coronaviruses.' Cepi is a global alliance leading efforts to finance and coordinate the development of the vaccine against COVID-19. It helps by filling any critical gaps in research, development, and innovation to advance the field of vaccines against infectious disease.

Coronaviruses have already caused two other recent epidemics in 2002-04 (SARS) and 2012 (MERS). In both epidemics, scientists had started working on vaccines, but these outbreaks were contained before the vaccines could be used. The company Moderna has repurposed its earlier work on the MERS virus carried out at the US National Institute of Allergy and Infectious Disease in Bethesda, Maryland. Another company, also based in Maryland, called Novavax has also used its earlier study of SARS, and its work on a vaccine, to develop one targeted for SARS-CoV-2, since these two viruses share around 80-90% of their genetic material.

Vaccines have traditionally worked on the principle of presenting a part or all of the pathogen to prompt the human immune system to protect itself by producing an antibody response to this pathogen. This would be in the form of inactivated virus particles or live attenuated low dose pathogens. Both methods have drawbacks: the live form may make its host ill by regaining some of its virulence, while the inactivated type might not offer the necessary degree of protection and may require higher or repeated doses.

More recent strategies involve isolating the genetic code from the protein spike found on the surface of SARS-CoV-2 (the 'crown'). This is then spliced into the genome of a bacterium or yeast to drive the altered microorganism into producing the protein. The theory is these proteins will then cause the body to produce an immune response against them. This type of vaccine is called 'recombinant'.

IS THERE A CONNECTION BETWEEN THE VACCINE FOR TUBERCULOSIS AND COVID-19 DEATHS?

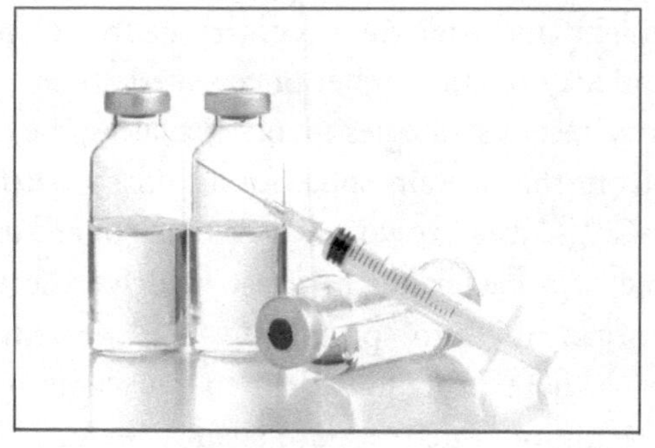

In 2011 a study was made to test the efficacy of Bacillus Calmette-Guérin (BCG) vaccinations in the prevention of acute upper respiratory infections in the elderly. This vaccine against tuberculosis is administered at birth in countries where the disease has historically been a danger, such as India. However, in some other countries, the BCG vaccine has not been introduced in the universal vaccination programme. In some countries, it may be an option for parents to consider, but not an enforced or heavily recommended one. Unfortunately, with the increase of anti-vaxxers, this might make uptake erratic. In poorer areas, where the relative danger may be higher, cost and availability may also come into play

The BCG vaccine has been around for around 100 years and is still the only vaccine in use to prevent tuberculosis (TB) in humans. Its efficacy has been a controversy since it is in the form of a live attenuated pathogen. This means that the particles of the bacterium Mycobacterium tuberculosis are present in the vaccine, but that they have been rendered inactive and unable to infect the body. The body thus uses these attenuated particles to form antibodies against the bacterium in its live form. Although it was found to be effective against some severe forms of TB, vaccines from different manufacturers seem to offer varying levels of protection. It keeps proving difficult to identify which strain should be used and further study on the genomics of the sub-strains is needed.

It is thought that the TB vaccine not only protects against the particular bacterium, but it also boosts the body's immune system against other pathogens such as viruses and parasites. The method by which this happens is not completely understood, but the vaccine may prepare the immune system to deal with an attack by pathogens other than Mycobacterium tuberculosis, offering a sort of shortcut when the body finds itself under attack.

In fact, it was found that countries that never enforced a universal BCG vaccine uptake were being hit harder by COVID-19, with a higher percentage of deaths per capita. For example, in Italy, where COVID-19 fatalities reached disastrous levels, BCG vaccine is only recommended to risk groups. Japan, where the number of reported deaths has so far been comparatively low, has a universal tuberculosis vaccine programme. This is despite delaying containment measures, which brought about a lot of criticism from other countries. Until the beginning of April, their death rate in Japan was around 2% compared to the 12.6% experienced in Italy.

The difference in the impact that COVID-19 has made between Western and Eastern Europe could also be explained in this way. A recent study by UK and US researchers which analysed data from 178 countries found that BCG vaccination incidence has made a tenfold difference in COVID-19 incidence as well as mortality. Countries of the former Soviet Union (USSR) had universal tuberculosis vaccination policies. Until the beginning of April, Germany, which had the Eastern part in the USSR until reunification in 1990, had lower cases per 100,000 people.

Of course, this information has many biases - finding positive cases depends on the number of tests being done in each country, and the style of contact tracing conducted. It does not include the number of asymptomatic patients who may not have been tested. Transparency in reporting is another important factor that should always be remembered. Culture always plays a role, in that the frequency and style of socialising and the hygiene methods practiced will make a difference when dealing with a pathogen spread via respiratory methods.

At the beginning of April, it was announced that medical research was being conducted to investigate if there may indeed be a correlation between BCG vaccine uptake and lower mortality rates due to COVID-19. These studies are using frontliners in at least 6 countries to run trials by administering the vaccine, although vaccines administered now may have a different effect to those used decades ago. While there may be several factors to keep in mind when examining the correlation between BCG vaccine uptake and mortality rate, the trend is conspicuous and warrants further analysis. With the whole world struggling to control this pandemic, and that it may be a while before a vaccine or treatment is confirmed, it may be worthwhile looking at whether the BCG vaccine could offer some sort of protection.

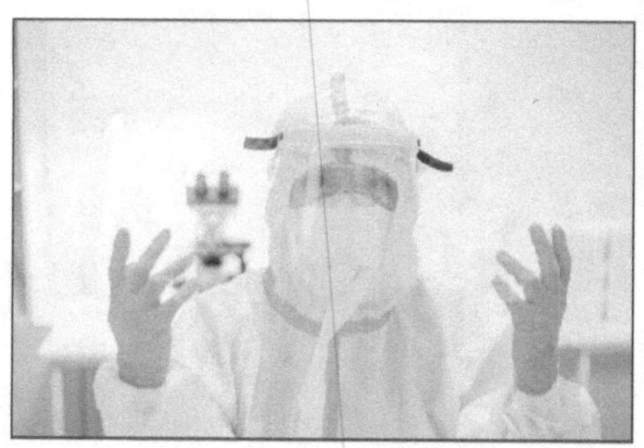

The coronavirus pandemic has highlighted the insufficiencies of healthcare systems in a stark fashion. It turns out that a costly market-based system is not equipped for researching, developing, and manufacturing medicines and vaccines in a timely manner. It is anticipated that it will take around 18 months before a vaccine can be available in an unrestricted manner. As seen with the previous outbreaks of MERS and SARS, this may be a case of too-little-too-late. The world has already lost too many lives to

COVID-19, and it may be a while before we have a real solution.

Crowdsourcing is a method by which connections with other people - in this case, experts such as epidemiologists, researchers, vaccine manufacturers and other scientists in laboratory testing and clinical trials - are used to access a large, relatively open, and often rapidly growing group of people to solve a task together.

The aim is to divide the work and share information and resources to achieve cumulative results more quickly. These medical and science experts pool in their knowledge and experience to get to solutions much faster than if they worked in separate teams. It is like tapping into a database of information but with a number of specifically-educated thinking minds at the end of it, all having the same aim and all putting their energy into finding a solution that works for all. This is the power of crowdsourcing, and during this pandemic, it may be the only thing with the possibility of curbing deaths and getting to solutions such as vaccines, proved cures, and even prophylaxis in a faster and safer way.

Teams usually in friendly - or not so friendly - competition with each other, and who possess some of the greatest minds and innovative technologies for this purpose, work together because it is a proven and intuitive way to get to the goal faster. In the interest of public health, should this be a permanent way of working? If governments are helping pharmaceutical industries in this state of emergencies, isn't it a good idea to always try to encourage the private sector to improve preparedness for such emergencies?

Essential health needs should be a priority, not

only during emergencies of this nature. However, the private sector has little incentive to work on counter-measures for future public health emergencies unless the profitability is assured, and unless they can worry less about patent abuses. The public sector may need to step in to offer these frameworks and assurances, for the good of all. During this pandemic, and in the immediate aftermath (whatever and whenever that may be), science may reign over politics and during this recognition the importance of such funding should be highlighted.

As Richard Hunt from the Department of Health in the US said of caring for the seriously ill COVID-19 patients: 'We are trying to fly the plane while we are building it'. Within months of doctors first encountering COVID-19 in patients in the Chinese city of Wuhan, medical staff from over 150 countries faced a growing number of such patients needing intensive care. Even though doctors treat patients with severe pneumonia frequently, the behaviour of the virus in the body does not follow the same patterns, and this makes it difficult to monitor the patients for deterioration or improvements.

The WHO has been crowdsourcing what hospitals around the world are learning about COVID-19. It has asked doctors to submit notes and to find information by analysing anonymous patient records that list procedures carried out, drugs prescribed, and outcomes. However, talking to doctors directly has seemed to work better, and this is over twice a week during a virtual gathering run by WHO. This means that knowledge can evolve quickly, and because of this, standards can be revised when needed.

A new website called COVID Near You was developed by the HealthMap team at the Harvard Medical School (HMS) and Boston Children's Hospital. COVID Near You encourages the people of the community to report their symptoms in real-time, identified by ZIP code only. This helps experts track the locations where COVID-19 is spreading or abating, and at which rate. This same tool was previously used for the flu. It relies on the community contributing in a quick and simple report kept anonymous except for location.

Another example of tapping into the collective wisdom is being conducted by NASA (National Aeronautics and Space Administration). NASA has issued a crowdsourcing call to its workforce to suggest innovative ways the agency and its resources can assist in the current ongoing battle against SARS-CoV-2. By identifying key problem areas and collaborating with the White House and other governmental groups participating in the response, NASA focused its efforts on the provision of personal protective equipment (PPE) and ventilating equipment, and means by which to track and monitor how the virus is transmitted and spread. Their decision was based on the identification of the most problematic areas at the time.

The focus on PPE could lead to an improvement on what we have - for example, self-sanitizing PPE that does not affect the filtration and safety of the equipment; techniques should be readily implementable, quick, effective, and not alter the function or fit even after several decontamination cycles. Ventilators should have a clean interface and be able to be produced rapidly. Designs should allow for quick regulatory approval for the fast delivery to public-private entities. Data analytics using NASA's most innovative equipment may allow experts to understand more about COVID-19 patterns and also about its economic, environmental, and societal impacts.

NASA announced a deadline of April 15th, 2020, to its staff in all areas and will be using the most viable ideas to further exploration. Any outcome, be it a product or a design, will result in an 'open source for any business or country to use', of course, depending on the kind of technology and resources needed. NASA has also contributed its efforts by lending its supercomputing capability and its artificial intelligence expertise to researchers during this difficult time. Ideas within NASA's mission could include telemedicine solutions and digital assistants for medical workers. With lessons learned in human space exploration, NASA could help us deal with social isolation and the new work-from-home model.

With the online video game Foldit, found at https://fold.it/, citizens can get involved in the work being done by scientists to find drugs that could help curb the spread of COVID-19. This crowdsourcing game lets the general public find ways to fold proteins. The unique shape of a particular protein and the way it folds gives it its particular properties. The game uses the collective mind to tackle the immense number of unique ways that even a small protein can be folded. Understanding which type of fold would be best in rendering it useful for understanding treatments for the virus takes a lot of time even when this is done by artificial intelligence - so the more people are doing it, the better are the chances of finding a solution.

Players can contribute to research by designing brand new proteins that could potentially treat or even prevent disease. Doing this in a gamified way that plays off people's creativity and competitiveness against each other takes advantage of the human brain's puzzle-solving and pattern-recognition skills. In turn, examining these skills and the way they are applied to the game, helps scientists teach computers (artificial intelligence) how to fold proteins faster and better.

RACISM AND PANDEMICS

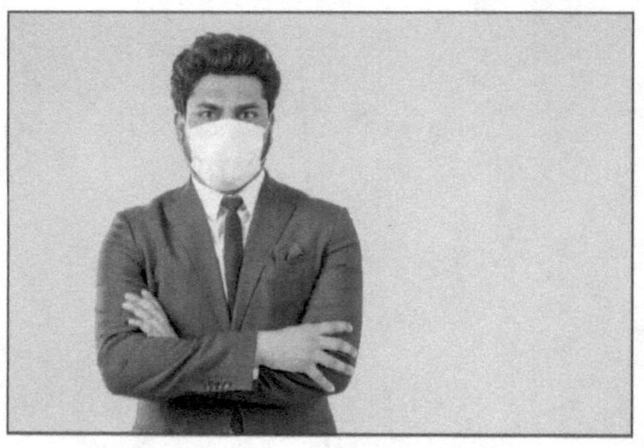

At the end of March, China issued a foreign visa ban effectively blocking all foreign nationals, even those married to a Chinese citizen. Even after lockdown measures are relaxed, there are likely to be more stringent measures in place. For example, the 10-year tourist visas normally distributed to Americans without too many restrictions might completely change in nature. New work visas may also require more scrutiny as anti-foreign and anti-Western sentiments seem to be on the rise during this time.

President Xi Jinping was reported to warn authorities against imported cases, although the Vice President of Foreign Affairs Luo Zhaohui announced that 9 out of 10 of China's new imported cases at the end of March were from those holding Chinese passports. In mid-April, as China prepared to fight off the second wave of COVID-19, the African community in Guangzhou suffered due to racist feelings that have been on the rise. Africans were unlawfully evicted from homes by their landlord for no good reason, and they have also been refused at hotels. Many had not travelled recently, nor had contact with COVID-positive patients. They were also treated in this way by the authorities who subjected them to random testing for COVID-19 and forced to stay in quarantine for 14 days, despite having no contact history or exhibiting any symptoms.

On the other side of the coin, discrimination against the Chinese or anyone with Asian features has gone up. As with most discrimination this is rooted in false impressions. According to an FBI report, Asian American communities were at an increased danger of suffering from racist acts and hate crimes during these times. Acts like these are not based on reason, so it wouldn't matter whether these Asian Americans had recently been abroad or come into contact with COVID-19 positive patients. Some of them may have never been to China in their life, despite their heritage. Incidents reported have included the refusal of service from a number of businesses, assault, and harassment. Some of this may have been incited by the vocabulary used by US President Donald Trump and his team when referring to the pandemic, e.g., 'China virus' or 'Wuhan virus'. Between the 28th January and the 24th

February, 1000 acts of xenophobia and racism were reported against Asian Americans; this coincides with the dates when the coronavirus began to spread in the U.S.

Stores run by Asians may also be feeling the brunt of this pandemic as people will tend to avoid such places in fear of contracting the infection from their service, or by coming into contact with their products. Activists in France made a sign that reads 'Coronavirus: It has made more people racist than sick.' The list of xenophobic, discriminatory acts, violence and racism against Chinese people, and any people that are Asian-like in descent or appearance, continues to grow around the world. This sentiment extends from individuals minding their own business to businesses trying to survive in an already difficult situation. Even Asian healthcare professionals have suffered this bad treatment as they try their hardest to help.

Cultural differences may further inflame racism even when acts are done with the best of intentions. For example, for Hong Kong natives wearing a mask during such a crisis, even if they live thousands of miles away from any Asian country, is a sign of respect and solidarity. The intention here is to protect the wearer and protect everyone around them. However, wearing a mask in New York in the days before the virus hit the state so hard may have looked suspicious and worrying. It may have attracted all the wrong kind of attention with people passing hurtful comments and even threats, and going out of their way to avoid the person.

With this seed growing in the back of people's minds, how difficult will it be to dislodge these ideas in the future?

This kind of scorn induced by a pathogen outbreak is not new. Disease causes uncertainty and fear and this can easily turn into discrimination, especially if the pathogen is new and not much is known about it. It has been stated repeatedly that stigma of this sort can be dangerous and sometimes more dangerous than the disease itself. With this in mind, the WHO tries to avoid choosing names for diseases that would encourage such preconceptions. A lesson was learned after naming Ebola as this name comes from the river in Congo, where the virus was first detected. There Africans were the target for discrimination and hate crimes. HIV and AIDS are examples of this fear and discrimination that, although not as rampant as in previous decades, still hangs around in the 21st century. Although HIV can only be transmitted via unprotected sexual intercourse or blood exchange (e.g., using the same needles to inject drugs), those who are HIV positive are often stigmatized and avoided, sometimes passively, but often through hate crimes.

WHAT WILL A POST-PANDEMIC WORLD BE LIKE?

A world in the midst of a pandemic feels surreal. It is difficult to know what lies ahead - and not just around the corner, but also in a future where the virus is no longer a huge new worry. Even though pandemic X was expected, and it was more of a matter of 'when' rather than 'if', nothing had prepared us for the real-life scenarios we have experienced and will continue to experience. Most speak of a 'new normal', and already there is reference to the way things were done 'pre-pandemic'. What will the future look like?

Information

One feature that distinguishes this pandemic from its predecessors is the prevalent use of social media and the ability to access all sorts of information from almost anywhere in the world. This, in itself, is part and parcel of the crisis. There is a lot of false informa-

tion and information that isn't helpful or is just specu-
lation. With people thinking they have become
knowledgeable because they're read a few articles on
the internet, or even had a complex thought, it is easy
to be led down a wrong path for obtaining facts. Due
to its constant developments, this pandemic has us
grappling to catch up with the 'latest'. In a struggle to
make sense of what's going on, it is only human nature
to seek to know more and understand. The problem is
that even experts do not always understand the way
this virus is working yet. Even those sharing snippets
of information on their social media timeline in a
benevolent manner may be doing more harm than
good if they have not fact-checked beforehand. Fact-
checking can be difficult and laborious and best left to
experts. Therefore this scenario begs the question -
who can we trust?

Politics vs Science

Scientists have warned us for years that such a
pandemic could happen and with a particular
emphasis on a respiratory pathogen. They have also
warned us about global warming and pollution, the
over-industrialisation of the world, the danger of
destroying animals' natural habitats and a myriad of
other issues largely ignored by politicians and governments. The pattern of too-little-too-late has been
magnified in the past few months. With this in mind,
who will we be listening to in the future? Experts or
heads of states?

And just like 9/11 and the 2008 financial crisis

changed the way we do things, we're in for another such ride. Scientists may need to devise new strategies in predicting the future using Artificial Intelligence (AI) technology, but this time the rest of the world might listen.

Interaction

When the worst of this is over, most people will respond with a sense of relief and a huge appreciation for the things they were not allowed to do for some time. They will want to see friends, to travel, and to enjoy leisure activities they had been prevented from doing. But will we have the same activities to go back to? Will we still eat out without thinking twice about where our meals are being made and by whom?

If it is possible to increase access to education, will we still require students to be in class for all of their lessons? Now that access is possible, will those who cannot physically attend have equal opportunities in a world where we have proven that online education works?

Business

Since the pandemic came on so fast and spread before businesses could prepare, it was very much a situation of sink or swim. Those who could adapt quickly, those with contingency plans, and those with savings stayed on top of the economy in crisis - or at least for a while with some sacrifices. Some businesses could quickly go online and have their workers do their jobs at home. Others changed the nature of their services and started delivering products rather than have people walk around their store. Certain sectors divided their staff into shifts so the interaction with different people would be limited.

However, workers in certain sectors such as tourism, hospitality, and entertainment, were suddenly 100% out of work. While some non-essential businesses could afford to maintain their staff on some sort of wage, most could not, and this was especially true in poorer areas or in small businesses that depended on their daily income to stay afloat. Workers who were fired or sent home on furlough still needed to pay rent and feed their families.

Those who could work from home faced different difficulties - for example, needing to take care of young children who were home from school, or having one computer to share between a couple and their children who needed to 'attend' school lessons online.

Some governments offered wages to those who lost work due to the pandemic, but the fear remains whether the money will get to the right people and whether this will be enough to feed their families.

Re-opening businesses may need to proceed in a staggered manner and people will need to be creative to keep their head above water in a situation where they may need to close again soon after they open. Certain scenarios may change for good. Is it necessary to travel for work if we've been successfully conducting meetings online? Is it wise to attract millions of people from all over the world to a conference? Should we use overcrowded means of transport? How dangerous is it to attend large events? Will concerts and festivals be a new breeding ground for the next pandemic? Will we eat out in restaurants as much as we used to? Who can we trust?

HAVE CHINA AND OTHER COUNTRIES MANIPULATED THEIR COVID-19 DATA?

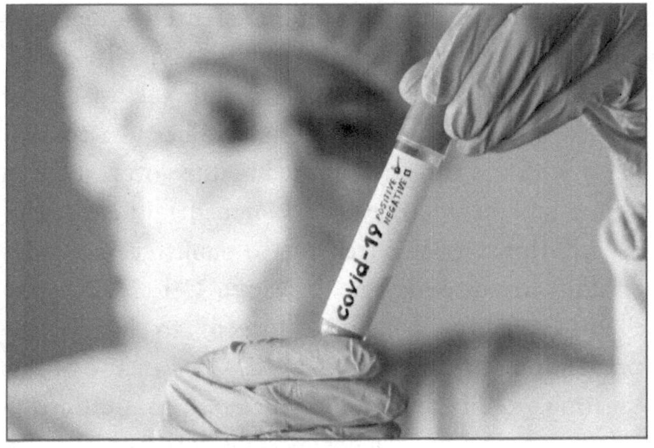

Between being the first to discover deaths caused by COVID-19, the first to sequence its genome, and the first to experience the outbreak - how much of China's data was available to the world, and how timely was it?

According to US officials, China kept the magnitude of the coronavirus outbreak in its country under wraps. This was reported in a classified document to the White House. Although the details of this document were not revealed, they divulged that it contained information about how China's reporting was 'intentionally incomplete'. The Chinese authorities also kept changing the goalposts of how reporting was conducted, sometimes omitting asymptomatic cases, then adding them again. In Hubei province, it was reported that thousands of urns appeared outside of funeral homes, and this did not tally with the number of deaths reported. Aside from concealing the truth from other nations, these discrepancies that later emerge as false, have also caused a mistrust of officials within the country itself.

Since the end of January 2020, Chinese researchers have published papers about COVID-19 in authoritative international medical journals. Through these, we could learn about the first cases of coronavirus infection and the milestones of an outbreak that later turned into a pandemic. These have been in controversy with the narrative offered by the government in China, and there has been a social media uproar in this regard. However, this freedom to publish came under scrutiny in a meeting held on March 25th, 2020, by the State Council's task force formed to handle the prevention and control of COVID-19. Because of this meeting, a directive was issued which outlined a vetting process for such papers. Before allowing for publication, papers would need a number of approvals - from the academic committees at universities, then to the science and technology department of the Education Ministry, and finally to the task force under the State Council. The directive states that "academic papers about tracing the origin of the virus must be strictly and tightly managed."

An anonymous Chinese researcher spoke to CNN

about his concerns that the Chinese government is trying to change the narrative about how and where the virus originated. One of China's leading universities, Fudan University in Shanghai, first published this on its website, and subsequently, the website was taken down. The China University of Geoscience in Wuhan also made a similar announcement and then removed the page. Other researchers stated that their papers published in February had not been placed under such scrutiny before publishing and thus, there is suspicion that perhaps some sensitive information had been published that placed the government of China in a difficult position. Parts of social media in China as well as the country's government, are questioning the origin of the virus and have repeatedly stressed that the exact origin has not been confirmed.

The transparency of reporting in the country where the virus originated is important because the response in the rest of the world was largely influenced by this initial information. Months later, seeing what happened in Italy and Spain, the information does not tally, and the extent to which the virus was spreading was suddenly much more alarming. For those countries hit very hard, emerging information was not of enough use, as it was too late to save the thousands of lives that could have been spared.

In mid-April, China changed the number of official deaths caused by the new coronavirus. On one day, they added 1290 deaths attributed to infection with COVID-19 in Wuhan, and another 325 confirmed cases. This declaration raises total deaths by a third to 3869, with the number of total cases reported being 50,333. With the death toll for Wuhan going from 2579 to 3869, the revised figure shows a 50% increase,

meaning they had previously hidden or left unde-
clared, half of the death toll. Officials said this
happened because in the overwhelming beginning
stages of the pandemic, people died at home and
medical staff were too overwhelmed taking care of
those they had a chance of saving to report the deaths.
Thus, they explained, there was a delay in the compila-
tion of final figures from various government and
private entities.

This wasn't the first time that such figures had
been altered by China, and these declarations came
amidst previous confusion, doubt, and mistrust across
the board. There were also discrepancies in the way
the Chinese measured their cases, omitting positive
cases that were symptomatic in their count. This made
comparisons with other countries across the world
difficult to make and renewed doubt in China's transparency during this crisis.

This takes us back to the start of the pandemic and
the crucial decisions made by China during that critical period. In light of the development that revealed
how the disease was really progressing, would other
countries have done things differently if the number of
deaths announced had been closer to the truth? Are we
to believe these new figures now?

An Associated Press report asserted that Chinese
officials played down what they knew was a very risky
situation when they got to know about the virus and
that they knew it might cause a pandemic. The impli-
cation is that when the outbreak started in Wuhan, the
country's leaders hid information available to them for
6 days - information that might have helped decrease
the impact of the virus in the rest of the world. These
claims are based on revelations from confidential

documents produced following a teleconference with China's National Health Commission. In one of these documents, one of China's top health experts warned that the viral outbreak 'is likely to develop into a major public health event.' He compared the challenge to the SARS outbreak, saying it was the most severe one since that time.

Key dates in January 2020 reveal a conflict in the information known in the inner circles and the actions being played out in public. In mid-January (14th), the clusters of cases suggested that human-to-human transmission was possible and maybe already happening. However, the severity of the situation continued to be downplayed in public on the 15th. Within 3 days after that, Wuhan was placed on lockdown. Meanwhile, with Wuhan being a major hub through which tens of thousands travel, the virus was spreading - supposedly beneath the radar. To make matters worse, this period of time coincided with the Chinese New Year, during which travel is popular with many. It is estimated that 5 million people left Wuhan, the epicentre of the COVID-19 outbreak, before the travel ban was put into place on the 23rd January 2020. In a paper titled 'Effect of non-pharmaceutical interventions for containing the COVID-19 outbreak in China' (Lai, Ruktanonchai, Zhou et al) it was revealed that had the containment methods been applied 7 days earlier in China, infections would have been decreased by up to two-thirds. The infections would have been cut by 95% if non-pharmaceutical interventions had been applied 3 weeks earlier.

In mid-April, USA President Trump decided to stop funding to the WHO, because he thought they had mishandled the coronavirus pandemic, especially pointing to the start of the outbreak in China. He claimed that the WHO had failed in its duties and had been promoting China's 'disinformation'. He insisted that the WHO was directly responsible for the magnitude of this pandemic and that they should have declared it a pandemic earlier in the year. This, despite him also publicly downplaying the coronavirus outbreak at the beginning of its spread to the US, and later declaring that he knew it would be a pandemic before the WHO declared a state of emergency.

Despite pointing at these mistakes made at the very start of the outbreak by the new coronavirus, a number of countries, and even states in the US, have made the same mistakes by adopting non-pharmaceutical interventions in a delayed manner. This has allowed the infection to spread rapidly because, as we saw, it would only take a slight delay for the numbers to rise rapidly.

This playing down of numbers to protect reputations of 'regimes' is suspected of a number of countries. Western officials have suspected this of Iran, Russia, Indonesia and North Korea, who are thought to have been under-counting. As of 12th April 2020, North Korea had not yet reported any cases, denying that COVID-19 has infected anyone in the country. As of the same date, Vietnam had only reported around 250 cases and no deaths, despite its having a long border with China. Nations of similar size, which are in the same area, had a much higher incidence of cases. This is despite both countries (Vietnam and North Korea) not having the resources of many nearby countries. While it is not possible to accurately measure community spread at this time, the low numbers reported stand behind a political agenda.

In some countries, it may be the lack of testing that makes a difference, but in others, the numbers may be altered purposely. The ability to 'flatten the curve' is a measure of the country's success in dealing with the crisis. If the goals are political, then it may be counter-intuitive to report real numbers and reveal how much the country has suffered.

Tracking the number of deaths caused by COVID-19 is tricky because the cause of death may not always be immediately apparent. Indirectly, people who have died due to other causes may have been saved if it wasn't for the healthcare system being so over-whelmed. They may have delayed treatment to avoid going to a doctor or to the hospital fearing getting infected, or because this help may have seemed less readily available, and so decreased their chance of survival. Patients dying in hospitals or at home of other complications would need further investigation to verify whether they were infected with SARS-CoV-2, and whether this was a contributing factor in their demise, and this created a delay in the way data is declared. These discrepancies are noted when looking at a measure called 'excess deaths'. That is, the number of deaths that occurred during a period of time as compared to the same period of time (in the same area) in previous years. By observing this historical data, we can see the gap between what we think are deaths by COVID-19 versus what may actually be the true number of people who fell victim to the virus, or to the lack of care.

When making these observations of mortality rates made by the national statistics office at the end of March, some noted that some countries (such as Italy) showed an excess of deaths double the official

COVID-19 count. One may presume that poorer countries are in an even worse situation, and we may never know exactly how many people have died of COVID-19 around the world. This is especially true of those countries where fewer tests are being conducted. Giorgio Gori, mayor of Bergamo, called the official death count 'the tip of the iceberg', acknowledging that many people were actually dying in their homes and not being counted in the official tally by the ministry of health. The true death toll in this region of Italy that was most severely hit may actually be 120% of the declared number.

In Spain, the overall deaths suggest that the true number may be 60% higher than the figures declared. In Britain, the death toll has been revised from 4300 to 6200 over 4 weeks in March 2020, but the records show that the actual excess deaths reached 7000. Except for New York, most states in the USA do not publish official death counts. This trend where the official death count must be extrapolated to include the actual number of deaths caused by COVID-19 was observed in New York, and one can presume this has been the same in other states too.

Political power also shows in how such news is reported. For example, in Vietnam, it is only the Minister of Health who can announce the number of COVID-19 positive cases found. Any other counts are considered unofficial, even if they are coming from hospitals and clinics, and these entities may also incur a penalty if they release such figures. The Communist Party in Vietnam (CPV) was just dealing with disquiet among its citizens in January 2020 following a deep-rooted land ownership dispute. Following an outcry against politicians on social media, extensive censorship was put in place. The outbreak of COVID-19 then gave the CPV an opportunity to boast about their effective model, which kept the cost as well as the number of victims low, with an aim to prove that it is prioritising the wellbeing of its people.

North Korea's institutions are in a similar position where reports of positive infections can easily be censored. However, on the 10th of March, the *Daily NK*, a South Korean online newspaper that focuses on North Korean issues, announced that the outbreak had killed 180 North Korean soldiers and that another 3700 were placed in quarantine in January and February. The newspaper also wrote that North Korean military leaders oversaw the sanitisation of areas where soldiers had been living. North Korea denies this information, but for the first time, they did mention economic losses sustained because of the virus outbreak. North Korea has also quarantined around 10,000 others, which may include around 380 foreigners, and has been releasing these as they showed no symptoms, despite saying that no cases had been found. Towards the end of March, they covertly asked leaders from other countries for help, including help with medical supplies needed to fight the new coronavirus. Worries persist that the situation might be out of control, or close to being so, and this is being hidden from the rest of the world

While it may be possible that the two countries may very well have managed to adopt measures to keep the virus at bay, in moves that have been much more successful than in other Asian countries, both have important political agendas that make the situation doubtful.

These discrepancies lead to a further lack of understanding of the global picture. If deaths are being hidden or disguised as having other causes, we may never know the exact extent of the damage that SARS-CoV-2 caused. Without a complete global picture, we may never know how much we could have done if we had known the full extent of this virus's power at an earlier stage.

Then there are the countries and leaders who take advantage of a bad situation to further their agenda. Take President of Russia Vladimir Putin, for example, who has set out to make the rest of the world believe that the new coronavirus is man-made and specifically man-made by the Americans in his wider effort to smear the West's reputation. He fulfills his aims by planting mistrust in the most important institutions whose purpose is to safeguard citizens' health, such as the CDC and the military. As the pandemic has made its way across the world, so has a tsunami of false information, in what the WHO termed the 'infodemic'. People are understandably confused and worried about the barrage of information they come across, and it's easy to play into this tension by disseminating conspiracy theories and fake news.

Via this disinformation, Putin's agents have previously sought to plant distrust in vaccinations. Despite the fact that during a televised meeting in 2018, he admonished parents who decided not to vaccinate their children, saying they are endangering their children's lives, he has worked to spur doubt in vaccines among the Americans. The threat of autism is still bounced around despite the fact that the theory has been disproved over and over again by experts. However, with these insidious messages being propagated by thousands of hired trolls over social media, especially Twitter, and with spokespersons being encouraged to insist on the misinformation, the message simply does not want to disappear for good. The coronavirus outbreak is being described as a designer weapon made to destroy China, or with the purpose of population control.

This is not the first time this method has been employed to plant mistrust in American institutions from within the country itself. The same happened during the Ebola outbreak and earlier than that during the HIV crisis. Both were described as pre-fabricated viruses with an agenda to use other populations as guinea pigs, or as racial weapons to kill black people.

WHEN WILL THINGS RETURN TO NORMAL?

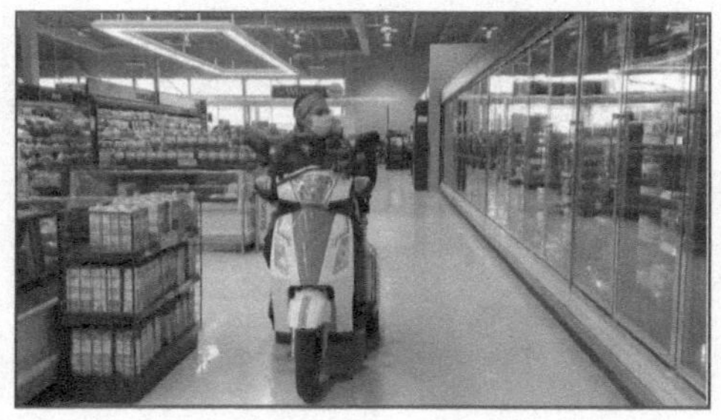

It is thought that when enough of the population, maybe around 60% or more of us, become resistant to COVID-19 it will be enough to curb the person-to-person transmission. No one knows if getting the infection, whether you are symptomatic or not, will make you resistant to further infection. When a pathogen attacks the body, the body sometimes has enough information to build antibodies specific towards that pathogen. This is done so that if the body encounters this same pathogen again, it would already have built a defence system to get rid of it in a faster and more efficient way, with less harm being done to the body. Vaccines work on this same principlebecause they induce the body to produce antibodies against the pathogen without causing the disease itself. Sometimes, as a side effect of taking a vaccine, there will be mild symptoms of the disease it is protecting you against.

Antibodies may be obtained from a component of the blood called serum from patients who have had the disease and have been cured. The message that the antibodies create in the body will stick around, especially when it comes to viruses. Sometimes, antibodies from serum are also obtained from animals to facilitate the detection of their presence in human serum. Some studies have shown there might be a relation between antibodies isolated from other coronaviruses such as those created during the SARS and MERS outbreaks. This means that the process may be accelerated as we learn more about what we can make use of, in terms of information that may already be available, during the COVID-19 pandemic.

The so-called 'herd immunity' or 'community immunity' is the principle on which vaccination works. Since a small portion of individuals cannot take a vaccine, and another portion of the population will be suffering from a compromised immune system, the general population will still carry an immunity if most persons are protected. This level varies with each infectious disease. For example, if a person contracts measles but is surrounded by people who are vaccinated against it, the disease will not be passed on to a new person. However, this only works if most people in the community are vaccinated. With measles, 19 out of every 20 people need to be vaccinated for there to be enough protection, and not even this is a guarantee of protection to those who are unvaccinated. As soon as the percentage of those who are vaccinated goes down, the danger of an outbreak becomes imminent. And so herd immunity does not give good protection for an individual, but vaccination does.

The return to 'normal' will probably be conducted in a staggered approach. Weighing out the options between possibly putting more people in danger and overwhelming the healthcare system, and protecting the economy as well as the mental health of those millions affected by lockdown measures is extremely difficult. The new coronavirus has spread so fast that experts have not had enough time to learn enough about it to be able to predict how the disease progresses and whether humans will be able to form the right antibodies for protection. Being given time, which is done by the methods employed to 'flatten the curve', is the best currency available. Countries' transparency on what is happening with their cases of COVID-19 is also crucial, but a means on which we, unfortunately, cannot rely in the current political scenario.

Asking people to stay at home and closing businesses deemed to be non-essential is aimed at slowing down the rate at which people contract COVID-19. It does not mean that the total number of positive patients will be decreased overall, but that the patients needing hospital care will be staggered to ensure that they can be treated. Some patients, of all ages and with any medical history, will need intensive care during their illness with COVID-19. Keeping the number of acute cases low and staggered decreases the chances of someone not being able to get the appropriate care. Even though some cases cannot be helped, especially if the patients are elderly and with underlying conditions, the majority of those with acute disease will survive if the appropriate and timely care is available. Meanwhile, while there are measures in place in order to slow down the spread, hospitals have the time to increase their capacity both in terms of beds and in equipment and staff needed for the increased demand. In most countries, this still leaves hospitals well under capacity for the rate at which the infection with SARS-CoV-2 spreads.

The needs of each geographical region differ, and even though data that is shared can be helpful, epidemiologists still study the needs of each particular region. For example, with the COVID-19, certain factors such as the demographics of the aging population, the density of the population and the presence of other compromising factors come into play. The intensity of the response, and the timing of each element in this response, need to directly correlate with the needs of a particular region.

By mid-April, most countries had gone through varying degrees of lockdown, shelter-in-place, or partial lockdown and physical distancing measures. Yet there were still no proven pharmaceutical measures nor effective vaccines on the horizon, despite the trials being done. With this dubious knowledge, and the world at a bizarre standstill, authorities needed to judge which measures were doing more harm than good. An important element remains the capacity of hospitals and of the care available in each country, state, or region. As numbers declined, and it is clear that hospitals can manage a substantial intake of patients, it may be time to relax measures in a controlled manner. Unfortunately, this may take a little bit of experimenting and the ability to go back and forth for a while until the results are clearer.

Late into April, when some countries seemed to have achieved peaks, and when cases had even started to decline in some areas, the talk turned to lifting restrictions. The WHO strongly suggested doing this in phases and Tedros Adhanom Ghebreyesus, director-general, held a virtual meeting in which he communicated this to the G20 leading global economies on the 19th of April 2020. He reiterated that countries were at different stages of the response and that they should look at easing restrictions not as the end of the pandemic, but as the beginning of a next phase in it. He emphasized that it was now the time for these countries to 'educate, engage and empower their people to prevent and respond rapidly to any resurgence', and that healthcare systems should remain as vigilant as ever to detect, test, isolate, care for every case, and analyse every possible transmission of contacts. A lifting of such measures is likely to cause a second wave of cases and resurgence of a burden to hospitals.

A study published in the beginning of April investigated the differences in the basic reproduction number R_0 occurring in different areas. This was estimated to be around 2-3 on average. However, variations were seen in some countries where a number of positive cases were first introduced via travel and then experienced fewer secondary cases than expected. This may indicate that not all symptomatic cases show the same degree of secondary transmission, which was also shown to be likely for past coronavirus outbreaks (SARS/MERS). There seems to be a variation on an individual level, meaning that some people may be superspreaders.

Superspreaders are unusually contagious people who are much more likely to spread the virus than other infected people are. This is thought to happen because of the way an individual's immune system works, making the person shed more of the virus into the environment when they cough or sneeze. If this is the case with COVID-19, it might be a key factor in preventing further spread. This study suggests that 80% of secondary infections could be caused by 10% of persons with COVID-19. These results make sense in the context of observed superspreading events during these first few months of the pandemic, with various countries having gone through the containment phase and the mitigation phase.

There is potential in investigating who these super-spreaders are, and how superspreading events affected transmission. This could lead to new strategies to protect people from these comparably infrequent superspreading events.

If any area should decide to relax the social distancing methods, strategies should be in place to test those with any (even light) symptoms, isolating those with symptoms and those with positive results, and doing thorough and fast contact tracing to estab-lish if any spreading has occurred. Behavioural change must be prompt, too, with self-quarantine becoming part of our lifestyle for the time being. Testing capaci-ties should remain strong and efficient until these risks for SARS-CoV-2 are around.

It might be a long time before we are not living with COVID-19. Our moves may need to have a finger on the pulse, considering the rate of transmission happening in the area, hospital capacities, testing capacity, and other population behaviour that may affect the notorious 'curve'. Self-quarantine should be tackled responsibly and seriously, and it should be supported by employers and governments to render it feasible.

Certain practices need to remain habits for the collective for good - hygiene practices, self-monitoring for illness, the protection of vulnerable individuals, funded access to prompt testing, and clinical follow-up of those who show symptoms just to name a few. High-risk environments should be monitored more closely, and any hint of illness should be examined promptly. A close watch needs to be kept on activities that cause people to congregate in groups. If work can be done remotely, then for some companies, this may be a good idea going forward.

This balancing act is the responsibility of all - because even when experts give guidelines, suggestions, and even orders, it is up to citizens to be careful and take precautionary measures when necessary. Of course, it is important to observe basic human needs and social constructs that keep society functioning well and humans mentally and physically healthy. Emphasis should be placed on data-driven decisions. Close monitoring and flexibility are crucial and this needs to be communicated efficiently in the face of fear and doubt.

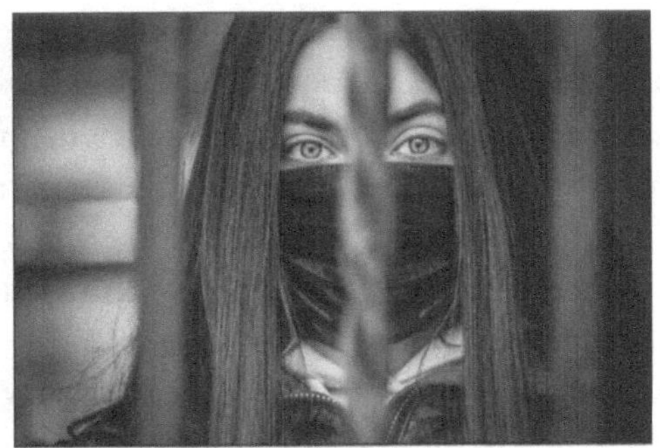

THE SECOND WAVE

At the end of April and the beginning of May, several countries and US states were planning to relax their physical distancing and lockdown measures. This was worrying the CDC, the WHO, the United Nations (UN) health agency, and other experts who think that it may be premature, especially when doing so without boosting healthcare first. In mid-April, when Austria, Denmark, Spain and Italy had already started to relax their lockdown measures, the WHO reiterated that bold tactics should be adopted against the virus. These were outlined as strategies to find, test, isolate, treat, and trace cases of potentially infected persons. They also highlighted that more should be done to discover those positive cases with mild or no symptoms, and trace contacts of such cases.

Even though some countries such as Spain and Italy had started to see a declaration of new positive cases, in others such as the UK and Turkey, cases were still on the increase. This caused a very 'mixed bag' scenario that made it difficult to decide on diminishing the restrictions. It showed that the transmission was not yet controlled. And with different countries having differing testing abilities, it was also difficult to know the true picture.

Equally important is making sure that the national health systems were supported and that healthcare workers were able to cope and getting enough rest. In some countries, the lack of PPE and the conditions of these workers were shocking; a second wave would only weaken what was already a system under too much pressure.

In countries where quarantine measures have been decreased, a second wave in the increase of positive cases occurred. On the one hand, countries cannot prolong the severe measures for too long due to economic losses and the mental health of their populations. On the other hand, easing the restrictions too soon could cause an even worse scenario where the decision needs to be reversed quickly and perhaps with drastic results.

Certain people have been hit harder than others, especially if they were already on the brink of poverty and got laid off or furloughed by their employers. Those living in overcrowded housing and conditions of lack of hygiene suddenly found themselves in horrific situations. It is impossible to be physically distant if you already live with too many people in one room.

In the US, where the pandemic has hit hard and has left more than 50,000 dead by the end of April, people are protesting against lockdown measures. These restrictions had been in place to different degrees for close to two months. The protestors have gathered in and outside of government buildings, disobeying physical distance measures as they do so. They have stopped traffic in city streets and held up signs questioning the requirement of continued quarantine measures, some even going as far as to call it a 'fake' crisis. President Trump has appeared to be on the side of the protestors in a series of stoking tweets such as 'Liberate Virginia!'.

POSSIBLE TREATMENTS AND ONGOING CLINICAL TRIALS

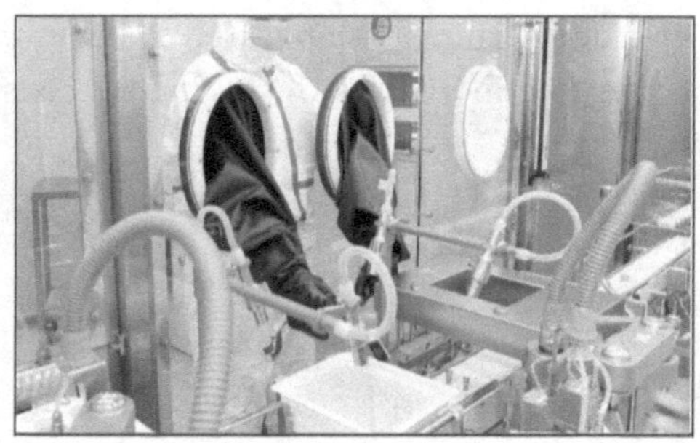

By the second half of April 2020, there were over 2,000,000 positive cases and more than 160,000 fatalities caused by COVID-19. The world was rushing to find a treatment, cure, or vaccine for this virus that seemed almost out of control. The medical world had never quite seen anything like this concerted effort, with large renowned companies joining forces and putting any differences aside in the race for finding the first proven treatment.

Within merely months of the disease spreading, researchers have set in motion more than 180 clinical trials ranging from those investigating Vitamin C, to repurposed antivirals, to immunomodulators, as well as antiparasitic drugs, combination therapies, and others. Since the majority of clinical trials never make it to the approval stage, it makes sense to go for several options at a stage where each passing day, week, and month makes a massive difference. It's also important to increase the chances at a point where we are continuously learning more about SARS-CoV-2, and what might work in treating it.

Some experts have criticised these efforts, claiming that they have been largely uncoordinated despite the best of intentions. The level of evidence for some drugs that have gone into trial has been low, already placing them in an unlikely position. This is not surprising since during a pandemic, time is not on our side, and scientists can get held back by the bureaucracy involved in coordinating efforts. It is a double-edged sword and a tricky dilemma - on the one hand, trying to go fast and, on the other, spending too much time on pre-trial research.

The WHO, together with other partners, started running a large international study of four treatment suggestions against COVID-19 called the Solidarity trial in March 2020. Its aim was to involve as many patients in as many countries as possible to jumpstart the search for treatment against COVID-19. The hope is to mitigate the risk of small trials not yielding satisfactory results and the strong evidence needed to establish and compare the relative performance of different methods. As of the first week of April 2020, over 90 countries were involved in the Solidarity trial, with the provision of simple methods to facilitate the participation of even the most burdened hospitals.

As of mid-April, there was not enough evidence to indicate the use of any treatments except for within the context of a clinical trial, and it was not recommended that hospitals or physicians around the world should attempt to prescribe any of these treatments of their own accord. The guidelines at this time supported only the use of standard treatments to alleviate symptoms when needed.

With no proven therapies having been established at the time of writing, the standard of treatment for COVID-19 symptomatic patients was supportive care. Fever and cough were treated with established medication. The care also included the use of either oxygen or mechanical ventilation, depending on the severity of the patient.

The WHO clinical trial - 'Solidarity'

The WHO, together with several countries participating, set out to test the efficacy of a number of treatments to try to find a cure for COVID-19 as quickly and efficiently as possible. This trial was going to be conducted in the hospitals of these countries, directly on infected patients, and in conjunction with any other standard care needed depending on the symptoms. It is hoped that by comparing untested treatments to each other, they will come closer to understanding which treatment proves to be right for the disease.

Dr. Tedros Adhanom Ghebreyesus, the Director-General of the World Health Organization, said of the trial, 'I'm glad that many countries have joined the

SOLIDARITY trial that will help us to move with speed and volume. The more countries that sign up to the SOLIDARITY trial and other large studies, the faster we will get results on which drugs work, and the more lives we will be able to save.

EIDD-2801

EIDD-2801 is an investigative new drug (IND) that the U.S. Food and Drug Administration (FDA) has authorised for use in COVID-19. On 13th April 2020, it was cleared for human testing. It acts as a broad-spectrum antiviral and has shown efficacy against influenza and Ebola, among other infections. It acts by preventing the replication of the virus SARS-CoV-2 in the body. In animal models, it has inhibited the viral replication of SARS-CoV-2 and MERS. The clinical trials with human patients are ongoing and have not yet yielded any definite results.

Remdesivir

Remdesivir is another antiviral originally used to treat Ebola and Marburg virus infections. It is a fluid administered intravenously (I.V. infusion) that has shown activity *in vitro* as well as *in vivo* against SARS-CoV-2. Even though it was originally formulated for Ebola, it did not prove as effective as other treatments at the time. Later it was used successfully in animal studies for other coronaviruses. On the 3rd of April, the European Medicines Agency (EMA) announced recommendations for using remdesivir for compassionate use, i.e., using an unapproved (or not yet approved) drug in a seriously ill patient when no other treatments are available.

Other antivirals such as favipiravir, oseltamivir, and ribavirin are also being investigated. Ribavirin is in clinical trials and was proposed for use alongside an interferon product to treat RNA viruses. Interferons are 'signaling' proteins produced by host cells to alert of the presence of viruses in the body. Favipiravir is available in China and Japan as a drug for influenza. It is also under clinical trial, and there have been no conclusive results so far.

Lopinavir-ritonavir (Kaletra)

This combination of drugs are used in HIV as protease inhibitors. They are usually used in conjunction with other antiretrovirals in the treatment of HIV infections. Lopinavir-ritonavir combination showed *in vitro* (in a lab, outside of a living organism) activity against SARS in a 2004 study. There are more than a dozen trials evaluating the efficacy of these drugs against placebo in the treatment of COVID-19. However, a randomized, controlled trial published in the *New England Journal of Medicine* revealed they were not found to show enough efficacy in patients with severe infection. Other trials being conducted should reveal results in late April 2020, in May 2020 and in July 2020, respectively.

.   .   .

Chloroquine and hydroxychloroquine

Chloroquine and hydroxychloroquine belong to a class of drugs called Quinolines, and they are used in the prevention and treatment of acute malaria. They are also used in the treatment of lupus and rheumatoid arthritis. These medicines have been under investigation and have shown some activity *in vitro* against coronaviruses when they were investigated during the MERS outbreak in 2012. It is thought that they work by changing the acidity on the surface of the cell, thus preventing the virus from invading it.

Some preliminary tests have been done using chloroquine and hydroxychloroquine alone or combined with an antibacterial drug azithromycin. It seemed that the combination therapy worked better to stop the spread of the infection, but this study was only conducted on a small sample of patients and was not deemed conclusive, despite the hype that arose about it. At the time of writing, this was not a recommended course of action due to the possible side effects that outweighed the potential for benefits.

Immunosuppressant Actemra (tocilizumab) and Kevzara (sarilumab)

The rationale behind the use of immunosuppressants is that the pathogenesis of the disease suggests a release of cytokines such as interleukin-6 (IL-6). Tocilizumab may reduce the mortality rate in severe or critical patients by acting as an IL-6 blocker. In studies conducted until the end of April, the overall certainty of this treatment succeeding was low, and there were concerns of the risk of bias since no control group was used. Some have suggested that its use may be most beneficial if it is given early in the disease. Sarilumab has been under study too, and some use has been anecdotally reported. It is thought to act in the same way by inhibiting IL-6.

Neutralizing antibodies against SARS-CoV-2

Based on the success of historical treatments for a number of infectious diseases, convalescent patient plasma or serum containing antibodies was proposed as a possible line of treatment. It is not yet understood whether getting infected with SARS-CoV-2 and recovering from the infection means that the patient will then be immune to getting the infection a second time. It is also not well understood what immunity to the coronavirus would look like.

Being immune to an infectious pathogen does not always mean you cannot contract it for life. Some have observed that antibody levels may wane over the years, and this has been the case with other coronaviruses. Losing antibodies years after infection does not necessarily mean that the patient becomes once again prone to the infection, as the 'blueprint' for making these antibodies for a specific pathogen may still be stored in the body. Unfortunately, not enough is known about how the immune system works to have clear answers at this point.

Following some clinical trials, no serious adverse

events were recorded, but the certainty of evidence remains low. The potential for side effects remains as there may be rare transfusion-associated risks in these procedures. Convalescent plasma has been used under the Emergency Investigational New Drug (eIND) application.

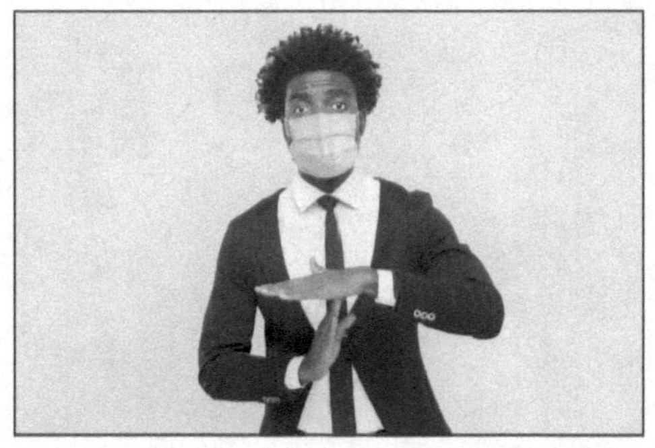

It's easy to see how a new virus that causes a pandemic in such a short span of time can be the breeding ground for fake news. Fake news is a name given to the reporting of false information or hoaxes in a deliberate manner. This information is spread via news or social media and can quickly become as widespread as the outbreak itself thanks to the internet. It can also be harmful in a similar manner. Even though the term 'fake news' has recently been used more often, the notion of dishonest campaigning has been around for hundreds of years under different names.

President Donald Trump, confined to the White House during quarantine, with his TV and his favourite news channels, made a lot of back and forth comments during the pandemic. As the leader of one of the biggest countries in the world, his words are scrutinised in a way he does not seem to take seriously. That is why he deemed it fit to accuse hospitals of squandering personal protective equipment and of hoarding ventilators.

Throughout January 2020, Mr. Trump downplayed the virus outbreak even though it had been rapidly spreading to various countries and was reported in at least 21 countries by the end of the month. That included the first case reported in the US, which was on the 20th of January. The patient was a 35-year-old man who had recently travelled to visit family in Wuhan, China. However, the American President thought it was all 'totally under control' and that 'it's one person coming in from China', repeating that 'it's going to be just fine.'

This also means that key steps that could have ensured that the United States was more prepared for the pandemic were not taken. For a while, travel continued in the usual manner and there were no provisions to increase the availability of life-saving equipment in the medical sector. Despite the public health data arriving from China, urgent warnings were largely ignored, and the US government was slow to act. Since those reassuring words were coming from the President, who was too busy worrying about his electoral popularity and possible impeachment, the

US lost time that would later turn out to be very bad news.

On February 10th, 11 days after the WHO declared the pandemic status, Trump spoke to thousands of supporters at a New Hampshire rally. He spoke of the virus 'miraculously' disappearing due to warmer weather in April. Yet in mid-March, he suddenly changed his tune and declared that he 'felt it was a pandemic long before it was called a pandemic'. It is no wonder then that his supporters are confused in this barrage of mixed messages and underplaying of events, and that they were driven to think of the very serious situation as a 'hoax'.

Confusing news from the authorities

Similar mixed messages have been delivered by several heads of countries who release guidelines and then create loopholes within these guidelines to be more popular with their constituency. The shorthand term 'infodemic' was coined during the SARS outbreak to represent the proliferation of information, including a barrage of fake data. It was now more relevant than ever as criminals and wrong-doers sought to use the outbreak as an opportunity to spread despair and division, and a way to take advantage of fear. This can curb a public health response that might otherwise have been effective; it creates confusion and harbours mistrust when we should be guided by science and facts.

When the spread of information is in the hands of those who don't realise how harmful their words may be, the result can be harmful in an immediate and long-term way. Take, for example, the fact that Donald Trump declared during a press conference at the beginning of April 2020 that he had his faith in the treatment with hydroxychloroquine, and there was nothing to lose in taking it, although there was no conclusive evidence for this. Elon Musk, tech entrepreneur and car manufacturer, also tweeted about chloroquine having no evidence.

These popular and newsworthy players get a lot of attention, and anything they say can be shared thousands of times and get misconstrued as a rightful endorsement, leading to false beliefs and more confusion. This also led to the hoarding of the antimalarial medicine in a way it was not available for those who really needed it. There were those who decided to try it in a move designed to keep them safe from infection with COVID-19, a move that led to some hospitalisations due to side effects of the same drug. The WHO has, at least until the end of April 2020, only recommended the use of hydroxychloroquine under clinical trial conditions.

In an unprecedented move, social media platforms Facebook and Twitter are working with WHO officials as 'mythbusters' to offset the spread of misinformation and spread of rumours via some statements, such as that the virus will not survive the hot weather, or that a large intake of garlic and ginger can prevent the virus. These companies are now acting as filters, to protect public health, by removing false information and preventing it from spreading more throughout their platforms.

It may seem obvious, but at a time of great tension and fear, a time when we don't understand what the future may hold, many of us become vulnerable to those who want to take advantage of the situation in a malicious manner. The public is being urged to get information only from trusted sources such as the World Health Organisation or the Centers for Disease Control and Prevention. They are also being cautioned against giving out personal information to anyone without official documentation, such as those who claim to be representing banks or other official agencies.

These pandemic times have also shown us how generous people can be and how they can come together during difficult times. Charitable acts have been experienced throughout the world - the hungry are being fed, the poor taken care of, the lonely entertained. Healthcare professionals are finally getting the recognition and respect they deserve. Other frontliners are respected for what they need to encounter in their jobs every day. We have rediscovered time and the need to cherish each other. We are spending more quality time with our family and communicating via new means. Artists have become even more creative, flourishing at a time when their work brings great solace. It may be time to see that our 'normal' is not the best place to go back to when this is finally 'over'.

This information was gathered during March and April 2020 and was deemed to be correct at the time of writing.

ABOUT THE AUTHOR

Miriam Calleja is a pharmacist and bilingual word-smith from Malta. She enjoys using her creative skills to explain complex ideas and make information more accessible to all through her medical writing.

Miriam has a keen interest in epidemiology, public health, and patient communications. She also teaches creative writing and works as an artist and poet. See more of her work at miriamcalleja.com

SOURCES

Cristiano Salata, Arianna Calistri, Cristina Parolin, Giorgio Palù, Coronaviruses: a paradigm of new emerging zoonotic diseases, *Pathogens and Disease*, Volume 77, Issue 9, December 2019, ftaa006, https://doi.org/10.1093/femspd/ftaa006

Fielding, B. What the latest coronavirus tells us about emerging new infections. MedicalXpress. 27th January 2020. https://medicalxpress.com/news/2020-01-latest-coronavirus-emerging-infections.html

Cui, J., Li, F. & Shi, Z. Origin and evolution of pathogenic coronaviruses. *Nat Rev Microbiol* 17, 181–192 (2019). https://doi.org/10.1038/s41579-018-0118-9

Zoonotic Diseases. Centers for Disease Control and Prevention. Last reviewed on 14th July 2017. https://www.cdc.gov/onehealth/basics/zoonotic-diseases.html

Coronavirus disease (COVID-19). COVID-19 | Corona Virus: Epidemiology, Pathophysiology, Diagnostics. Ninja Nerd Science. Accessed at: https://www.youtube.com/watch?v=PWzbArPgo-o

Goudarzi, S. Lessons from past outbreaks could help fight the coronavirus pandemic. Scientific American. March 23rd 2020. Accessed at: https://www.scientificamerican.com/article/lessons-from-past-outbreaks-could-help-fight-the-coronavirus-pandemic1/

The Deadliest Flu: The Complete Story of the Discovery and Reconstruction of the 1918 Pandemic Virus. By Douglas Jordan with contributions from Dr. Terrence Tumpey and Barbara Jester.
https://www.cdc.gov/flu/pandemic-resources/reconstruction-1918-virus.html

That Discomfort You're Feeling Is Grief by Scott Berinato
March 23, 2020
https://hbr.org/2020/03/that-discomfort-youre-feeling-is-grief?fbclid=IwAR35_lZ8_xajIcqad-GfMTT6_Hcp_ytepXFah30uvVNMHnbri4RB6GmVPC4

Kreuder Johnson, C., Hitchens, P. L., Smiley Evans, T., Goldstein, T., Thomas, K., Clements, A., Joly, D. O., Wolfe, N. D., Daszak, P., Karesh, W. B., & Mazet, J. K. (2015). Spillover and pandemic properties of zoonotic viruses with high host plasticity. *Scientific reports, 5*, 14830. https://doi.org/10.1038/srep14830

Heffernan, J. M., Smith, R. J., & Wahl, L. M. (2005). Perspectives on the basic reproductive ratio. *Journal of the Royal Society, Interface, 2*(4), 281–293. https://doi.org/10.1098/rsif.2005.0042

Zimmer, C. Welcome to the Virosphere. The New York Times. March 24, 2020.

Coronavirus vaccine: when will it be ready? 25 March 2020   https://www.theguardian.com/world/2020/mar/25/coronavirus-vaccine-when-will-it-be-ready-trials-cure-immunisation

Singh, SK. Middle East Respiratory Syndrome Virus Pathogenesis. Semin Respir Crit Care Med 2016. DOI: 10.1055/s-0036-1584796

Strochlic, N. Champine, RD. How some cities 'flattened the curve' during the 1918 flu pandemic. National Geographic. 27th March 2020. Accessed at: https://www.nationalgeographic.com/history/2020/03/how-cities-flattened-curve-1918-spanish-flu-pandemic-coronavirus/

Laguipo, ABB. How does COVID-19 coronavirus compare to the 1918 Spanish flu? News Medical Life Sciences. March 9th 2020. Accessed at: https://www.news-medical.net/news/20200309/How-does-COVID-19-coronavirus-compare-to-the-1918-Spanish-flu.aspx

Goudarzi, S. Lessons from Past Outbreaks Could Help Fight the Coronavirus Pandemic. Scientific American.

March 23rd 2020. Accessed at: https://www.scientificamerican.com/article/lessons-from-past-outbreaks-could-help-fight-the-coronavirus-pandemic1/

Ho, MS. Severe Acute Respiratory Syndrome (SARS). Section II: Pathogens, Part E: Viral Infections. Chapter 59.
Peiris, J., Guan, Y. & Yuen, K. Severe acute respiratory syndrome. *Nat Med* **10,** S88–S97 (2004). https://doi.org/10.1038/nm1143

Global Preparedness Monitoring Board. A world at risk: annual report on global preparedness for health emergencies. Geneva: World Health Organization; 2019. Licence: CC BY-NC-SA 3.0 IGO.

Use Of Cloth Coverings To Help Slow Spread Of COVID-19. Centers for Disease Control and Prevention. 4th April 2020. Accessed at: https://www.cdc.gov/coronavirus/2019-ncov/prevent-getting-sick/diy-cloth-face-coverings.html

Covid-19: risk factors for severe disease and death. BMJ 2020; 368 26 March 2020. Doi: https://doi.org/10.1136/bmj.m1198

Bendix, A. Secon, H. Men are dying from the coronavirus at higher rates than women around the world. Here are scientists' best ideas as to why. Business Insider. March 30th 2020. Accessed at: https://www.businessinsider.com/why-more-men-die-from-coronavirus-than-women-2020-3

Hindson, J. COVID-19: faecal–oral transmission?. Nat Rev Gastroenterol Hepatol (2020). https://doi.org/10.1038/s41575-020-0295-7

Wardhana1, Datau EA, Sultana A, Mandang VV, Jim E. The efficacy of Bacillus Calmette-Guerin vaccinations for the prevention of acute upper respiratory tract infection in the elderly. Accessed at: http://www.inaactamedica.org/archives/2011/21979284.pdf

Coronavirus Will Change the World Permanently. Here's How. Politico Magazine. 19th March 2020. Accessed at: https://www.politico.com/news/magazine/2020/03/19/coronavirus-effect-economy-life-society-analysis-covid-135579

Crowdsourcing to fight COVID-19. The Economist. March 26th 2020. Accessed at: https://www.economist.com/international/2020/03/26/crowdsourcing-to-fight-covid-19

Etherington, D. NASA issues agency-wide crowdsourcing call for ideas around COVID-19 response. Techcrunch.com. 1st April 2020. Accessed at: https://techcrunch.com/2020/04/01/nasa-issues-agency-wide-crowdsourcing-call-for-ideas-around-covid-19-response/

"BCG Vaccination Policies Make a Ten Times Difference in Covid-19 Incidence, Mortality: New Study." The Economic Times. Accessed April 3, 2020. https://m.economictimes.com/industry/healthcare/biotech/healthcare/nations-without-bcg-vaccination-saw-higher-cases/articleshow/74956201.cms.

Wadhams, N. Jacobs, J. China Concealed Extent of Virus Outbreak, U.S. Intelligence Says. 1st April 2020. Bloomberg. Accessed at: https://www.bloomberg.com/news/articles/2020-04-01/china-concealed-extent-of-virus-outbreak-u-s-intelligence-says

Palmer, J. What to make of China's coronavirus figures? Foreign Policy. April 1st 2020. Accessed at: https://foreignpolicy.com/2020/04/01/china-coronavirus-official-figures-underreporting-pandemic-response-xi-jinping/

Gan, N. Hu, C. Beijing tightens grip over coronavirus research, amid US-China row on virus origin. CNN. April 13th 2020. Accessed at: https://edition.cnn.com/2020/04/12/asia/china-coronavirus-research-restrictions-intl-hnk/index.html

Broad, WJ. Putin's Long War Against American Science. The New York Times. April 13th 20202. Accessed at: https://nyti.ms/2Xvbdhn

Billings, K. Racist Acts Surge Against Asian Americans During Coronavirus Pandemic. International Business Times. 27th March 2020. Accessed at: https://www.ibtimes.com/racist-acts-surge-against-asian-americans-during-coronavirus-pandemic-2948149

Coronavirus Will Change the World Permanently. Here's How. Politico Magazine. March 19th 2020. Accessed at: https://www.politico.com/news/magazine/2020/03/19/coronavirus-effect-economy-life-society-analysis-covid-135579

Griffiths, J. Jiang, S. Wuhan officials have revised the city's coronavirus death toll up by 50%. CNN. 17th April 2020. Accessed at: https://edition.cnn.com/2020/04/17/asia/china-wuhan-coronavirus-death-toll-intl-hnk/index.html

Griffiths, J. AP report claims China knew of pandemic danger in Wuhan even as officials downplayed risk of virus. CNN, 17th April 2020. Accessed at: https://edition.cnn.com/2020/04/16/asia/china-wuhan-coronavirus-ap-intl-hnk/index.html

Shengjie Lai*, Nick W Ruktanonchai*, Liangcai Zhou, Olivia Prosper, Wei Luo, Jessica R Floyd, Amy Wesolowski, Mauricio Santillana, Chi Zhang, Xiangjun Du, Hongjie Yu, and Andrew J Tatem. Effect of non-pharmaceutical interventions for containing the COVID-19 outbreak in China. March 13th 2020. Accessed at: https://doi.org/10.1101/2020.03.03.20029843

Craven, J. COVID-19 therapeutics tracker. Regulatory Affairs Professionals Society. April 16th 2020. Accessed at: https://www.raps.org/news-and-articles/news-articles/2020/3/covid-19-therapeutics-tracker

Auwaerter, P. Coronavirus COVID-19 (SARS-CoV-2). John Hopkins Medicine. ABX Guide. April 21st 2020. Accessed at: https://www.hopkinsguides.com/hopkins/view/Johns_Hopkins_ABX_Guide/540747/all/Coronavirus_COVID_19__SARS_CoV_2=

Tracking covid-19 excess deaths across countries. The Economist. April 16th 2020. Accessed at: https://www.economist.com/graphic-detail/2020/04/17/coronavirus-infections-have-peaked-in-much-of-the-rich-world

Endo A, Centre for the Mathematical Modelling of Infectious Diseases COVID-19 Working Group, Abbott S *et al.* Estimating the overdispersion in COVID-19 transmission using outbreak sizes outside China [version 1; peer review: awaiting peer review]. *Wellcome Open Res* 2020, **5**:67 (https://doi.org/10.12688/wellcomeopenres.15842.1)

Cher, A. Countries risk second wave of coronavirus infections by easing restrictions too early, says expert. CNBC. April 14th 2020. Accessed at: https://www.cnbc.com/2020/04/14/countries-risk-second-wave-of-coronavirus-infections-by-easing-restrictions-too-early-says-expert.html

Relaxing lockdowns without boosting care could lead to new COVID spike: WHO. United Nations. April 15th 2020. Accessed at: https://news.un.org/en/story/2020/04/1061782

Ellis, R. Maxouris, C. McLaughlin, EC. Azad, A. As states grapple with reopening their economies Trump says part of Georgia's plan is 'just too soon'. April 23rd 2020. Accessed at: https://edition.cnn.com/2020/04/22/health/us-coronavirus-wednesday/index.html

Department of Global Communications. UN tackles

'infodemic' of misinformation and cybercrime in COVID-19 crisis. Accessed at: https://www.un.org/en/un-coronavirus-communications-team/un-tackling-%E2%80%98infodemic%E2%80%99-misinformation-and-cybercrime-covid-19

'infodemic' of misinformation and cybercrime in COVID-19 crisis. Accessed at: https://www.un.org/en/un-coronavirus-communications-team/un-tackling-%E2%80%98infodemic%E2%80%99-misinformation-and-cybercrime-covid-19